COMMUNITY OCCUPATIONAL THERAPY WITH MENTALLY HANDICAPPED ADULTS

FORTHCOMING TITLES

THERAPY IN PRACTICE SERIES

Edited by Jo Campling

This series of books is aimed at 'therapists' concerned with rehabilitation in a very broad sense. The intended audience particularly includes occupational therapists, physiotherapists and speech therapists, but many titles will also be of interest to nurses, psychologists, medical staff, social workers, teachers or volunteer workers. Some volumes are interdisciplinary, others are aimed at one particular profession. All titles will be comprehensive but concise, and practical but with due reference to relevant theory and evidence. They are not research monographs but focus on professional practice, and will be of value to both students and qualified personnel.

Community Occupational Therapy with Mentally Handicapped Adults

DEBBIE ISAAC

CHAPMAN AND HALL
LONDON • NEW YORK • TOKYO • MELBOURNE • MADRAS

UK	Chapman and Hall, 11 New Fetter Lane, London EC4P 4EE
USA	Chapman and Hall, 29 West 35th Street, New York NY10001
JAPAN	Chapman and Hall Japan, Thomson Publishing Japan, Hirakawacho Nemoto Building, 7F, 1-7-11 Hirakawa-cho, Chiyoda-ku, Tokyo 102
AUSTRALIA	Chapman and Hall Australia, Thomas Nelson Australia, 480 La Trobe Street, PO Box 4725, Melbourne 3000
INDIA	Chapman and Hall India, R. Sheshadri, 32 Second Main Road, CIT East, Madras 600 035

First edition 1990

© 1990 Debbie Isaac

Typeset in 10/12pt Times by Mayhew Typesetting, Bristol
Printed in Great Britain by St Edmundsbury Press Ltd,
Bury St Edmunds, Suffolk

ISBN 0 412 32720 1 (PB)

British Library Cataloguing in Publication Data

Isaac, Debbie
Community occupational therapy with mentally handicapped adults. – (Therapy in practice).
1. Mentally handicapped persons. Rehabilitation
I. Title II. Series
362.38
ISBN 0 412 32720 1

Library of Congress Cataloging-in-Publication Data

Isaac, Debbie, 1959–
Community occupational therapy with mentally handicapped adults / Debbie Isaac. – 1st ed.
p. cm. – (Therapy in practice series: 16)
Includes bibliographical references.
ISBN 0 412 32720 1 (pbk.)
1. Occupational therapy. 2. Mentally ill – Rehabilitation.
3. Mentally handicapped – Rehabilitation. 4. Community mental health services. I. Title. II. Series.
[DNLM: 1. Community Mental Health Services. 2. Mental Disorders – rehabilitation. 3. Mental Retardation – rehabilitation. 4. Occupational Therapy.   WM 450.4.02 I73c]
RC487.I8   1990
362.2′2 – dc20
DNLM/DLC
for Library of Congress   90-1456
                                                            CIP

Contents

Acknowledgements

I was lucky enough to be spotted by Jo Campling at the Annual
BAOT Conference in Newcastle-on-Tyne in 1986 whilst doing a
presentation with Anne Lodge, which is how the idea to write a
book came about. The source of inspiration was my 2½-year
experience in the North Southward Community Mental Handicap
Team (CMHT). The job itself was enormously satisfying, but very
stressful at times. I was enabled to stay there because of the tremendous support and guidance I received from my District Therapist,
Stephanie Correia, and the Head OT at Grove Park Hospital, Wendy
Close. Without them this book would never have been written.

Many people contributed indirectly by way of discussion and
experiences at work – colleagues at North Southwark CMHT, from
community groups and other occupational therapists. These include
Nick Bouras, Nan Carle, Barbara Chambers, Janet Chambers, Linda
Clarke, Sharon Collins, Lillian Davis, Win Fleming, Beverly
Harker, Rita Hartington, Theresa Heggarty, Geraldine Holt, Val
Huffington, Anne Lodge, Chandra McGowen, Dee Napier, Barley
Oliver, Sarah Organ, Sally Pennington, Lindy Pogue, Julie Rivers,
Nadia Simpson, Howard Slater, Claire Tester, Smithy Thiru and
Chris Vicerman, the team of support workers at North Southwark
CMHT, and occupational therapy staff at Guy's Hospital, New
Cross Hospital and Southwark Social Services.

Of practical contributions to the book, Janet Chambers was
responsible for compiling the original Day Services Questionnaire
(see Appendix 2) for the North Southwark team, and additions have
since been made with the help of Chris Mackie. The guidelines for
architects (Table 5.1) were based on a document written with
Theresa Heggarty, Beverly Harker and Katrina Cooper. The outline
for operational policies (Chapter 5) is based on the operational policy
format used by Sharon Collins and her staff at the Southwark Mental
Handicap Consortium. Thanks go to Hyde and Southbank and
Habinteg Housing Associations and Peter Mischcon and Associates,
for allowing the reproduction of architects' plans.

My husband, David Tofler, has been encouraging and supportive
throughout the writing process and contributed to the content and
layout of Chapters 7 and 9. My mother, Golda Isaac, has helped
with her unstinting domestic support.

For assistance with the computer, thanks go to Gideon Gild and
Harold Zwier, and for typing, to Geelong Mobile, Sheila Gray and
Ruth Tofler.

Preface

The philosophy of normalization and promotion of the plight of children and adults with mental handicaps has drawn more public attention in recent years. Governments in a number of countries have embarked upon policies involving the closure of institutions, movement of people with mental handicaps back into the community, and development of community-orientated programmes, although their reasons for this may be economically, rather than ideologically, motivated. Occupational therapists have moved into the community, along with other health professionals, in order to set up community services for people with mental handicaps.

My own experience of working in a multidisciplinary team in Central London for 2½ years, helping adults with mental handicaps to move out of an institution, has been a source of motivation to write this book. The amount of written material available on the occupational therapy approach to resettlement and de-institutionalization is limited, in comparison with the massive amount of information written by, and for, other practitioners. Additionally, the number of texts written by and for occupational therapists with this client group are few. Despite excellent support from OT colleagues, I experienced considerable frustration trying to define and perform my role, not helped by a shortage of texts to draw on.

The topics included in the book are varied, and serve to highlight important issues that OTs working in the community, in general, and with this client group particularly, should address. The intention is that this book be used as a guide, to indicate pertinent issues for therapists to consider, and indicate useful approaches and resources. In some instances, a range of opinions are detailed, leaving the reader to draw his/her own conclusions. A large number of papers, programmes and texts have been cited to support various opinions, but also in the hope that the interested reader will refer to them for a more detailed discussion of the topic concerned.

The terminology used to describe the client group are 'adults with a mental handicap'. There are a variety of terms used in practice – 'intellectual disability', 'mental retardation', 'learning disorders', and 'developmental disability', to name a few. As 'mental handicap' was the term most used whilst I worked in London, and because the book is based largely on my experience there, I have used it as my term to describe the client group.

Some of the references used date back to the 1930s, although the majority are from recent publications. Early references have been included because of their highly relevant and illustrative value. Where possible, I have attempted to demonstrate the natural development of practices with people with mental handicaps. (For example, many of the theories and approaches to group and individual therapy with people with a mental handicap had their origins in the 1930s and '40s).

As there are several texts cited that may not be available in the bookshops, an address list of the organizations that print them has been included.

Debbie Isaac

Useful addresses

The purpose of the address list is to enable the reader to obtain references from organizations, as listed below, whose publications do not ordinarily appear in bookshops. Some of these groups also run courses, which will be helpful to O.T.'s living in the United Kingdom only.

Architectural Press, 9 Queen Anne's Gate, London, SW1

British Institute of Mental Handicap (BIMH), Wolverhampton Road, Kidderminster, Worcs., DY10 3PP

Campaign for Mentally Handicapped People, 12a Maddox Street, London, W1R 9PL

Centre on Environment for the Handicapped (CEH), 126 Albert Street, London, NW1

Department of Health and Social Security, Alexander Fleming House, Elephant and Castle, London, SE1

Department of the Environment, 2 Marsham Street, London, SW1P 3EB

Disabled Living Foundation, 380–384 Harrow Road, London, W9 2HU

Disabled Living Foundation (Sales) Ltd, Book House, 45 East Hill, London, SW18 2QZ

London Housing Consortium — West Group, 112 Uxbridge Road, Hayes, Middlesex, UB4 8JX

National Unit for Psychiatric Research and Development (NURPD), Lewisham Hospital, London, SE13

NFER-NELSON, Darville House, 2 Oxford Road East, Windsor, Berkshire, England, SL4 1DF

NIMROD The White Houses, 40–42 Cowbridge Road, East Canton, Cardiff, Wales, CF1 9DU

Phoebe Caldwell, Hortham Hospital, Almondsbury, Bristol, BS12 4JN

Royal Institute of British Architects, 66 Portland Place, London, W1N 4AD

Southwark Mental Handicap Consortium, Cambridge House, 131 Camberwell Road, London, SE5 OHF

Spastics Society of Victoria, 135 Inkerman Road, St. Kilda, Victoria, Australia 3142

1

Community occupational therapy and the multidisciplinary team

Much has been written about the historical background and framework from which the profession of occupational therapy has emerged, and upon which basic tenets of occupational therapy practice rest today (e.g. Englehardt, 1977; Reed, 1984; Lyons, 1985). Without going into detailed analysis of these texts and others, the philosophical basis for the profession can be summarized by the following beliefs:

1. That all people, including those with physical, psychological and intellectual disabilities, are capable of achieving some level of independence in their daily lives, from the most basic tasks such as feeding oneself, to more complex ones, such as participating in a particular leisure activity unaided; and
2. That people need to see themselves as purposeful, productive and achieving in order to stay alive.

The task for the occupational therapist (OT) therefore, is to enable all clients referred to pursue these goals, and for the therapist to 'tailor' his/her intervention to the particular needs of the individual concerned. Therefore, the range of tasks and role that the OT adopts in a particular facility will vary and will be largely dependent on the types of problems presented by the clientele.

THE OCCUPATIONAL THERAPIST IN THE COMMUNITY

Several authors have examined the range of tasks taken on by OTs in community (i.e. non-hospital) settings, based in clients' homes or local community facilities (Brough and Hooyveld, 1978; Kewish, 1979; Milne and Mathews, 1979; Blundy and Prevezer, 1986).

Brough and Hooyveld note tasks undertaken by OTs working from a community mental health centre in a residential part of London to encompass: (a) retraining in home management; (b) resettlement into purposeful occupation/employment; (c) relaxation and social skills training; and (d) encouraging the development of personal and creative outlets.

Kewish describes her work with people with psychiatric and psychological difficulties in an industrial area of Melbourne with a high proportion of migrants and notes OT tasks to include: (a) assessment of new clients; (b) individual and group work, e.g. assertiveness training, adolescent awareness identity group; (c) setting up self-help groups; (d) developing a toy-making co-operative; and (e) locating volunteers to be involved in a variety of tasks.

The work undertaken by OTs in local government described by Milne and Matthews is very broad and covers: (a) the provision of advice to clients and employers with regard to resources available to people/workers with disabilities; (b) the issuing of aids and organiza-tion of housing adaptations; (c) provision of specialist service to disabled children, adolescents, the elderly and those with a mental handicap; and (d) keeping abreast of new developments, teaching students and speaking to community groups.

In a description of their work in community teams in Central London, providing a service to adults with mental and physical handicaps, Blundy and Prevezer note OT tasks to include: (a) work-ing with clients to improve motor, feeding, communication, personal hygiene, cooking and social skills in group and individual settings; (b) assessing clients in order to set up programmes in the home, residential or day settings of for future placement; (c) promoting independence and integration in leisure pursuits; (d) counselling clients and their families; (e) participation in case conferences, plan-ning and policy meetings, talks to community groups; and (f) taking on OT students for placements.

The variety of tasks in which the OTs working in this setting become involved has been attested to in recent surveys (Special Interest Group – Mental Handicap, 1987; Newman, Donoghue and Rees, 1988). It has also been observed that the nature of the diffi-culties that people with mental handicaps present require the OT to take a very broad approach to his/her work (Anstice and Bowden, 1985).

In all of these situations mentioned, the tasks taken on by the therapist were largely a response to the populations they were serving. The following factors also played a role in moulding their jobs:

1. Tasks common to all professionals in the facility, such as the assessment of new clients (Kewish, 1979) or participation in planning and policy meetings (Blundy and Prevezer, 1986);
2. The stage of team development, e.g. whether the OT was starting out at the beginning of the team's formation or whether he/she was coming in at a time when there has been a vacancy for some time. Spashett (1981) notes that nurses have moved into the implementation of rehabilitation programmes in the absence of OTs in hospital settings. It could be inappropriate for an incoming OT to 'take over' groups run by other professionals in such a situation; he/she would have to consider carefully what areas were more immediately open for exploration, with a view to long-term involvement in activity groups;
3. Expectations of other team members – this can influence the number and type of referrals directed to the OT. In a survey of expectations of health team personnel towards OTs in the Guy's district in London, Correia (1981) noted that OTs were generally well recognized but were under-utilized, as their colleagues were not fully aware of the range of skills that the OTs could offer. The importance of OTs enlightening colleagues as to their range of skills, writing more extensive notes in the files of their clients and promoting opportunities for postgraduate training for themselves is emphasized. Blundy and Prevezer (1986) and Kewish (1979) note the time spent with colleagues discussing training backgrounds, skills and interests as vital to establishing their roles and understanding their colleagues, too;
4. Degree of role blurring – this relates to the extent to which people define the boundaries of their 'team' role and individual 'disciplinary' role and is connected to the tasks which they share in common. Krupinski and Lippman (1984) describe a situation where the maintenance of 'blurred roles' and 'generalist' philosophy in a community health centre ultimately led to divisions amongst the staff group. The establishment of role boundaries is aided by frequent communication with colleagues and by carving out a niche of very specialised work. For the OT, this could be the provision and organization of aids and adaptations. This is particularly important as occupational therapy overlaps in some areas with other paramedicals, e.g. with speech therapy in feeding, with psychology in the process of

skills training and with physiotherapy in recreational activities;

5. Team leadership – the style of leadership and decision-making can also affect the type of tasks the OT takes on. The chairing of meetings, writing of letters and regular 'link' visits to outside agencies are 'leadership' tasks often shared by team members, in an effort to maintain a democratic process (Blundy and Prevezer, 1986). The progress that leaderless groups can make is somewhat dubious, and in fact, despite all efforts, often a leader emerges on the basis of a task or group dynamics e.g. the administrator who co-ordinates incoming correspondence, the secretary who organizes meetings or the person who shouts the loudest at a meeting. Invariably there is a need for good chairing, and when in that position, one needs to establish the length of time of the meeting, set the agenda, keep the meeting to time, allow each person to have their say, be able to sum up a discussion and steer the group towards a decision. Wherever possible, leaderless teams need to agree on a basic format of chairing;

6. Team base – the location of the team base can be a great influence on one's style of working. It is a common experience of health teams to be obliged to work in cramped offices with little privacy, limited opportunities to interview clients privately or work quietly. This can oblige the OT to seek alternative venues for work with clients that is not suitably done in the home, or spend most time away from the office. This invariably means time is spent organizing other facilities. If the service is new, or not conveniently or obviously located, it may mean that the OT, like his/her colleagues, will need to spend time informing the community about the service's existence and location;

7. Management directives – these will strongly influence the sphere of work that teams engage in. Many mental handicap teams have been set up in the UK with the express purpose of facilitating the movement of mentally handicapped adults from long-stay hospitals back into the community. This has required occupational therapists to spend time at the hospital concerned, assessing and getting to know clients as against working in the community to develop various self-help programmes. Other pressures in this situation include deadlines for hospital closure and financial cutbacks;

8. The 'responsibility' entailed in community work. It is not an uncommon experience of OTs working in the community to find that they are the only field worker involved with a client/family. It may be impossible to involve other agencies because of long

waiting lists or because other workers may have been rejected by the client. This places a weighty responsibility on the worker concerned, particularly if the client has multiple problems, e.g. psychiatric difficulties in addition to mental handicap. This puts the onus on the therapist to maintain a wide level of reading on a range of physical and psychological difficulties, and to maintain, seek and refer to other agencies as appropriate. For further discussion on the influences on practitioners in a community mental handicap team, see Simon (1981) and McGrath (1988).

WORKING OUT YOUR OWN ROLE AND JOB DESCRIPTION

This can be an awesome task, particularly if coming into an established team where there has been little or no occupational therapy input. In such a situation there are several tasks that the OT must tackle before settling upon a 'role' and/or job description.

1. Try to assess what the major needs of the clients are, e.g. the need for aids, appliances, skills training, a support group for carers. This is an on-going process but it is useful to define a few specific tasks initially;
2. Establish what resources are presently available in the community, e.g. other occupational therapists, community facilities, voluntary organizations;
3. If there are resources, how accessible are they to consumers, i.e. how difficult is it to refer a client to the resource/centre; is it accessible to people with physical disabiities?
4. What resources are there in the team and how do team members perceive their roles and tasks?
5. How do team members perceive your role and potential tasks as an occupational therapist?
6. What are the management directives with regard to the team's role and priorities?
7. Are there criteria for client referrals? This needs to be very firm, if one is not to be obliged to take one's clients inappropriately.
8. What are the administrative procedures in the office e.g. procedure for client referrals or client assessments?
9. What are the overall goals of the team?
10. Who lives in the community, e.g. ethnic groups, the elderly?

11. Find out what are the facilities for transportation, recreation and housing for your particular client group.

Having gone through the above process, the therapist should have gathered hard-core information about existing community services and the 'indigenous' population. It is vital to have sufficient time (at least 3–4 weeks) to look around the community when first posted to a community job. Liaison with community groups and organizations needs to be maintained once the therapist becomes involved in client work and other administrative aspects of the job.

Community liaison can be overwhelming but can be managed by prioritizing the organizations most relevant to the therapist and his/her clients. Regular meetings can be established accordingly, whether they be every two months or twice a year (see Chapter 2). One should aim to spend up to 10% of work-time in community liaison work. Other reasons for such work include informing the community about occupational therapy, collecting referrals, being aware of community developments and avoiding duplication of work.

Job description

Having viewed the community at close quarters, the OT needs to check that his/her initial job description concurs with the community's needs. If this is not the case, the job description should be revised with agreement from management; if the therapist does not have a job description, he/she will need to write one.

Job descriptions are important for:

1. Informing others in the organization about the tasks you are going to do;
2. Establishing work boundaries with colleagues and minimizing 'role blurring';
3. Keeping 'on task' to comply with management directives and client needs;
4. Giving structure to your work.

Job descriptions should be reviewed every six months to ensure that they comply with changing client and organizational needs.

For the OT working in a multidisciplinary team distinguishing between OT tasks and tasks shared in common with other team members is vital. For OT tasks reference needs to be made to: (a) assessment type (e.g. activities of daily living, ADL); (b) how the OT will carry out the result of any assessment (e.g. devise specific training techniques, work with parents/care staff, run groups, individual work, etc); (c) liaison with other OTs; (d) own professional development; (e) teaching/resource role to other staff, students the community, etc; and (f) some general remarks about client work, e.g. acceptance of referrals, attendance at case conferences, doing relevant paperwork, liaising with co-workers, etc.

Additionally, the OT will need to blend into the job description specific tasks that may relate to the overall brief of the team. For example if the team is to be involved in moving clients from one long-stay institution to the community, reference should be made to OT involvement in the establishment and refurbishing of housing to meet clients' needs.

Team tasks also need to be noted in the job description, and again will be dependent on the team style. This could include chairing of meetings, involvement in the planning and development of the service, liaison with community agencies, public relations etc.

The previous discussion on the variety of activities that OTs working in the community in different settings can involve themselves in (Brough and Hooyveld 1978; Kewish, 1979; Milne and Matthews, 1979; Blundy and Prevezer, 1986) indicate a good deal of overlap between clinical areas.

The skills and tasks required of OTs with clients with physical and mental handicaps are much the same as for OTs working in mental health clinics and community centres. Community OTs need to be versed in a wide variety of skills, to have access to super-vision and support from experienced therapists and specialists, plus opportunities for further training. The onus is on the managers of therapists in the community to ensure these facilities are made accessible to their staff in order to:

1. Maintain a high standard of practice amongst community staff;
2. Give the staff the resources they need to perform the job;
3. Keep staff enthusiastic;
4. Give staff 'time-out' from the stresses of community work (see below).

WORK STRESS IN THE COMMUNITY

Much has been written about the stresses suffered by workers in the human service professions and their susceptibility to burnout – 'a syndrome of physical and emotional exhaustion, involving the development of negative self-concept, negative job attitudes and loss of concern and feeling for clients' (Pines and Maslach, 1978, p.233). Health workers have been identified as particularly at risk from work stress and burnout (Cunnick and Smith, 1977; Pines and Maslach, 1978; Lamb, 1979; Scholem and Perlman, 1979; Freudenberger and Richelson, 1980; Hegarty, 1987; Mayou, 1987; Illot, 1988).

The findings of these researchers can be applied to occupational therapists engaged in field work. Sturgess and Poulsen (1983) summarize the causes of burnout as related to:

1. Personality and lifestyle characteristics of the health professional, e.g. the overcommitted worker whose life outside the job gives little satisfaction, the authoritarian worker who feels that no-one else can do the job as well;
2. Nature and severity of clients' problems, i.e. the poorer the prognosis of the client, the higher the incidence of burnout amongst staff caring for the client;
3. Demands of the work situation, e.g. long hours, heavy case loads, low pay, insufficient time for client contact, poor institutional support.

There is some literature which looks at the incidence of work stress and burnout amongst OTs. Findings include the following:

1. That OTs feel secure within their own numbers but are less secure in a team setting (Phil and Spiers 1977); working in a team setting may produce role misunderstanding and conflict which Kahn (1978) found to be a potent source of burnout;
2. OTs working with acute psychiatric, geriatric or mentally handicapped clients have less job satisfaction and sense of personal accomplishment than therapists working in general hospital or, paediatric settings (Sturgess and Poulsen, 1983); the researchers attribute this to the differing job charateristics (e.g. a very high patient:therapist ratio for the job);
3. Burnout amongst OTs is related to poor preparation for working with people with chronic conditions (Burnett-Beaulieu, 1982);
4. OT managers tend to have more negative attitudes towards service recipients and score higher on an emotional – exhaustion

scale than do staff therapists (Brollier *et al.*, 1986). The researchers suggested that the OT managers may be more susceptible to burnout because of insufficient training in management skills and having to cope with the dual role of administrative and client-centred work. They also suggested that the managers may have retreated into management because they were already burnt out.

To date, there is no empirical research on OTs working in the community, although one must suspect that they are just as vulnerable to burnout and work stress as hospital-based therapists. Indeed, they have additional difficulties to deal with, some common stressors being: working in isolation from other OTs, not having equipment or a place to assess clients, no technician on hand, travelling, clients spread out over a wide patch, and heavy traffic.

Despite this gloomy picture, several practical tasks can help to monitor work stress in the community, as in other settings.

Supervision

Smith (1978) describes a programme of psychotherapy supervision for OTs working in psychiatric units, where weekly sessions are used to discuss problems with clients, groups or other work-related issues. For community OTs, Ibbotson (1983) suggests sessions of 1–1½ hours are held every 3–4 weeks with the senior person in charge. She suggests that the sessions require structuring and could be based on: (a) review of new cases, in terms of immediate and long-term plans and resources, and focus on the wider aspects of handicap, such as the impact on families, appropriate use of agencies, writing of reports, saying 'no' to clients and interview techniques, or (b) agenda set by supervisor and therapist based on a wide range of issues, set at the beginning of each meeting.

Structured supervision sessions are indeed advantageous for several reasons:

1. Feedback can be given to the therapist on a regular basis;
2. It can help the therapist to structure her work and control her case-load;
3. It is an opportunity for the manager and therapist to keep in touch with what is happening in the field and for the therapist to keep in touch with more administrative developments;
4. It gives the therapist a chance to 'let off steam' and explore alternative approaches to clients and staff in a neutral setting.

9

Supervision needs to be regular and have structure. Although Ibbotson (1983) suggests every three to four weeks, it may be more effective if this is done more frequently for less time, e.g. once a fortnight for an hour. Supervision should be a matter of negotiation, depending on the needs and experience of the therapist.

A *psychotherapy* supervisor need not be an occupational therapist, and needs to be chosen on the basis of work expertise (Smith, 1978). This should be the guide to follow for the community OT engaged in individual psychotherapy or group work. However, aside from this, it is preferable to seek supervision from an OT manager. For further discussion on supervision within the OT profession, see Munroe (1988).

Job-related responses

Various manoeuvres related to the structure and nature of the job can be employed to monitor work stress. Staff can be regularly rotated through the most stressful areas and time structured at work to have time away from direct client contact, e.g. a set time for administrative duties, report writing, etc. Training needs of staff should be identified and opportunities given to attend courses. OT specialists need to be identified and accessed to field workers. It may be useful to employ a group approach in order to share work problems and client load in addition to individual supervision, although this could be problematic in a fragmented team. Seeking out other community therapists and exchanging ideas and experiences can provide perspective and support in one's own situation. Maintaining work hours is a simple way to limit work load.

Personal responses

Discharging feelings about work can be directed through physical exercise and distance and by regular vacations. Learning one's own personal limits can set a marker for what one is prepared to take on – but this is more easily said than done.

For further discussion on responses to work stress within the OT profession, see Craik (1988) and Cox (1988).

WORKING IN MULTIDISCIPLINARY TEAMS

Multidisciplinary teamwork is a common structure in health services. As well as providing an opportunity to work closely with colleagues from other disciplines it can be an extremely torrid and stressful experience.

Barriers to team functioning

Barriers to effective multidisciplinary team functioning have been listed by Pollock (1986) to include:

1. Differences in the management lines, career structures and conditions of work team members;
2. Differing organizational demands on each profession can mean unequal sharing of responsibility and decision-making, e.g. demands on OTs to run workshops and supervize students could mean less time spent with individual clients, leaving nurses on the ward to cope with them;
3. Professional background of team leaders and the styles of leadership and decision-making;
4. Role confusion through failing to identify professional and personal contributions that could be made by team members;
5. Failure to clarify overlap of skills and role boundaries, e.g. speech therapists, occupational therapists and physiotherapists can all be involved in facilitating independence in eating – each needs to agree on who will do what, and what the boundaries will be;
6. Differences in gender, e.g. with regard to decision-making, women tend to go for consensus rather than autocratic decisions;
7. Differing perceptions about rehabilitation and approach to clients due to differences in training;
8. Personality and cultural backgrounds of team members.

In addition to the above, poor office conditions with little privacy and a lot of activity (e.g. telephones buzzing, typewriters clacking, people going in and out) can be an irritating and demoralizing intrusion into work practice and team functioning.

The workings of multidisciplinary teams can also be viewed in terms of the 'group process'. Tuckman (1965) and Tuckman and Jensen (1977) describe the life cycle of the group in terms of: (a) forming – getting acquainted, questioning the group purpose, trying to work

11

out what behaviour is appropriate; (b) storming – development of power struggles, testing other members and leader, clarifying group talk; (c) norming – establishing methods to achieve task, roles emerging in group both formal (e.g. chairperson) and social (e.g. the humorist, the troublemaker etc); (d) performing – activity to achieve task, high level of cohesion amongst group; and (e) adjourning – evaluating task, break up of group, group members dealing with this impending loss.

Many of the difficulties that occur in teams can be seen in a group dynamics context. Groups/teams will move backwards and forwards between the stages depending on what is going on.

Scapegoating

Scapegoating is often used as a device to avoid being in the spotlight when group members don't want to focus on their own conflicts, perceptions and feelings (Fielding, 1982). For example, overworked team members may pick on someone who fails to write in a file on one occasion.

Change in group membership

Reversion to a behaviour pattern of an earlier stage of development can be triggered by a crisis, such as a change in group membership (Crawley, 1978). 'Testing-out' of incoming members is associated with the 'storming' phase. Group members may resent the new-comer's intrusion into the intimacy of the group or fearful that he/she may introduce new 'rules' that would upset the *status quo*. 'Testing out' can take the form 'by-passing' the newcomer, by the discussion of past events of which he/she is ignorant, or by attack using aggressive interpretations (in a T-group setting) (Fielding, 1982). For example, any constructive remarks made by a newcomer may be ignored or ridiculed.

Group cohesion

Group cohesion and progression through the various stages of group development is dependent on how well the group members can relate in the same phase at the same time. A group will only proceed through the stages if members are willing to let it grow (Charrier, 1972). For example, a group cannot progress to carrying out a task (norming and performing) if it is bogged down in power struggles or trying to define the task.

Group leadership

Leaders in groups, whether designated or self-appointed, give group members a focal point for locating and resolving issues of control and initiative. Without leadership, the group will find it difficult to make decisions and decide upon appropriate group action for achieving goals (Crawley, 1979).

Common ploys used by leaderless groups to 'maintain democracy' and prevent the emergence of a natural leader include the establishment of unrealistically high requirements of agreement amongst members, the absence of a structure to deal with the resolution of conflicts, and the institution of a rotating chairperson (Crawley, 1979).

The notion of a leaderless group is a myth, as some form of self-appointed, undesignated leadership, perhaps in the form of a clique, will emerge. Cliques are a definite barrier to group cohesiveness (Charrier, 1972). They are a feature of the 'storming' phase and are a means by which power over the group can be wielded in the absence of an identified leader. In addition to verbal interaction, body language may also be employed by the clique in standing over the group, e.g. members of a clique sitting together in a meeting.

Observing a particular group process can give one an understanding of, and perspective on the situation and may lend one to consider various options towards a solution.

Reducing the barriers in team work

The existence of barriers and difficult group dynamics in a team not only affects the ability of the team to progress and achieve goals, but can also have an impact on those outside the team. For example, in the absence of a leader, outside agencies may not know who to contact for a referral. The signing of general correspondence by different team members (as described by Blundy and Prevezer (1986)) may be confusing for agencies receiving the letters. Changeable external representation of a team does not bode well for public relations, for those attempting to present a professional and organized image. It is therefore desirable for both team functioning and external image to overcome the barriers which can block team functioning.

Holt and Oliver (1989) describe ways to enhance team functioning and reduce stress in community mental handicap teams. In particular they identify: (a) induction training for new team members, (b) joint planning and writing of clear operational policies and (c) closer involvement of management in the work of CMHT's in achieving these goals.

Organizational barriers

The structure of an organization may be difficult to break down, but some group cohesion can be gained by team members airing their frustrations and anger about the organization together (Pollock, 1986). However, there is a risk of being tricked into the 'Ain't it Awful' game (Berne, 1964), at which point the therapeutic aspects-sharing begin to get lost. The team might also consider who in the organization could be targeted for directing their grievances. If a poor relationship exists with management, the team should consider methods to improve communication, such as regular meetings with management, and the sharing of information, such as reports or minutes of meetings. Establishing rules for confidentiality in meetings may encourage group cohesion if team members feel they can present their views in confidence (Pollock, 1986).

In the presence of outside organizational disarray, it is vital for team cohesion to establish a sense of order from within. Administrative procedures for the ordering of equipment, petty cash, record keeping, structuring of meetings, chairing and minute-taking need to be clarified, in addition to leadership of the team (permanent or temporary, such as rotating chairperson) and what it entails.

A key to good team cohesion is a clear policy on the acceptance of referrals. A common problem experienced by workers in the mental handicap field are those clients who suffer from additional psychiatric difficulties. The question is: which service is most appropriate for the client's present problems? A constructive way to look at referrals when they arrive, is to try and establish what the primary problem is, and what service can best deal with it.

In order to separate out the needs of clients being referred, and exert control over a flood of referrals, a set of criteria must be found for the acceptance of a client to a service.

Example: Acceptance of clients into a community service for mentally and physically handicapped adults was defined by:

- age (clients had to be over the age of 18 years);
- evidence of mental handicap, such as an IQ score;
- attendance at a special school;
- (in)ability to perform various daily tasks, such as dressing, bathing, shopping and money handling;
- mental handicap being the *primary* problem for the client;
- other services involved with the client, such as a specialist social worker for adults with mental handicaps.

One should not be obliged to accept clients on the basis of absence of other services. This indicates an inability for the service/therapist to set boundaries and is a causative agent of burnout.

Lack of agreement on the acceptance of referrals can cause disunity in a team. In order to promote consistent working pattern and group cohesion, a policy on the acceptance of referrals must be agreed upon.

Role conflict

Time needs to be laid aside for team members to openly exchange views on their professional roles (Pollock, 1986). Given that the atmosphere created by 'team work' can be rather intense, with not only tasks to achieve, but also an interpersonal dynamics to contend with, teams should consider having a session with a facilitator on a regular basis (e.g. once a fortnight for an hour) to enable sharing, and allow the expression of angry feelings in a structured group setting. This is particularly important in the absence of a permanent leader.

The minimization of role conflict can be established by a clear boundary as laid out in a job description (see earlier in this chapter).

Tasks to be shared by all must be clearly established. A key-worker system whereby each client is allocated to a worker who co-ordinates and organizes the client's care, is an effective way to ensure that work is not duplicated and defines a structure for client care whereby workers can broaden their roles (Pollock, 1986). It is important that this is done in the context of members' job descriptions.

Differing training backgrounds

The division inherent in a team as caused by different training backgrounds of professionals could be minimized by more shared training at an undergraduate level (Pollock, 1986). Whilst this is an idealistic solution on a practical level, the introduction of joint training sessions 'on-the-job' for all team members may provide opportunities for common learning, as well as for swapping different perceptions about rehabilitation, work issues, etc.

Personality differences

Giving respect to others' views is the key to avoiding polarization of opinions in teams (Pollock, 1986). Teams need to be cohesive enough to tolerate disagreement before attempting to clarify tasks and goals.

Social outings

Informal social contact outside work provides an opportunity for team members to meet under more relaxed circumstances. Efforts should be made not to 'talk shop' and to discover the other dimensions of colleagues. Some people will prefer to maintain a professional profile and may be isolated from others wanting to be more sociable. The development of a social clique may be destructive to the group in the long term (Pollock, 1986). It may require the more socially aloof person to step out of his/her role in order to 'balance' the process.

CONCLUSION

The occupational therapist in the community has a lot to contend with and some of the challenges have been noted.

However, in order to progress, he/she must retain an optimistic outlook, and together with management, look at practical ways for making the job more manageable, satisfying and enriching. Working in a multidisciplinary team has its disadvantages, but the implementation of structures and honest communication with colleagues can enable the tackling of interesting and challenging projects.

2

Institution to community

The philosophy of 'normalization' expounded by Wolfensberger (1972) and the United Nations Declaration of the Rights of Mentally Handicapped Persons (1971) have undoubtedly done such to raise the consciousness of communities and governments as to the inadequacy of institutional service provision to meet the needs of people with mental handicaps.

Normalization promotes the recognition of this group of people as valued members of society with the same needs and rights for determining their lives as 'normal' people.

RESEARCH IN SUPPORT OF COMMUNITY PROGRAMMES

Whilst recognizing that the adoption of policies advocating the establishment of community programmes for people with mental handicaps may have an element of political expediency, it is worthwhile noting some of the findings of researchers which support the idea.

Quality of care and development of skills

Russell (1985) notes the work of researchers in the 1950s and 1960s who demonstrated that so-called 'ineducable' people had the potential to acquire new skills and perform tasks and that such development could be hastened by programmes and accommodation taking place in a small homely environment (Tizzard, 1960; 1964).

In a literature search with regard to quality of care given to people with mental handicaps, Balla (1976) notes that quality of care is determined by the practices of carers rather than the kind of housing.

Care practices in community-based facilities tend to be more orientated towards the needs of the individual (McCormick, Balla and Zigler, 1975), promote organizational effectiveness (Klaber, 1969), and a more nurturing atmosphere (Harris *et al.*, 1974). Tizzard (1964) observed that caretaking and educational practices of staff orientated towards individual clients in small units, promoted behavioural growth.

Genuine cognitive growth has been observed in clients who are mentally handicapped, following movement to smaller community-based residential settings from large institutions (Shroeder and Henes, 1976). Behaviour gains in personal and community self-sufficiency have been observed as a function of residential proximity to community services (Eyman, Demaine and Lei, 1979). Further to this, Locker, Rao and Weddell (1984), found that small community-based hostels provided an excellent environment in which people with mental handicaps could acquire the social and personal care skills necessary for more independent living. Kleinberg and Galligan (1983) suggest that skills are within the client's repertoire, but that the environment and therapeutic (as against custodial) staff approach encourages skill usage.

A close examination of the impact of ordinary housing on four mentally handicapped individuals (living in a staffed house) noted improvements in their quality of life, with regard to activities engaged in, and contact with people (Evans *et al.*, 1987). A move to the community has also been observed to facilitate levels of adaptive behaviour, activity, social interaction and contact with the community (Allen, 1989).

Individual case studies and descriptions of group homes illustrate one impact of community living on people with mental and physical handicaps in a very personal and graphic way (McDevitt *et al.*, 1978; Hunt and Smith; 1982; Meyers, 1985; Walters, 1985; Halpern, Close and Nelson, 1986; Johnson and Wallace, 1986; Bratt and Johnston, 1988; Day, 1988).

Family contact

Beside improvement in the quality of life, another major argument in favour of small community-based facilities is that the individual has greater access to his/her friends and family (Balla, 1976; de Kock *et al.*, 1988). Parents appear to be more likely to visit their children if they are living in smaller units (Klaber, 1969). Individuals residing in a group home are more likely to go to their family homes for visits and see their friends than those living in long-stay institutions (Campbell, 1968). Frequency of visits has been found to be related to the distance to be travelled by relatives as well as the age of the resident concerned (Dalgleish, 1986). Dalgleish notes that it is likely that parents of older, ex-residents may be frail and unable to travel or have lost contact with their children through the course of time. Family contact appears to be a major factor in determining integration into the community by ex-residents of long-stay institutions (Schalock and Lilley, 1986).

Aside from research findings, it would appear that living in the community can enlarge the range of social contacts and life experiences that people with mental handicaps can have, although this may largely depend on the practices of any care staff involved.

Financial considerations

Proponents of community care have also argued for it on the basis that it is cheaper. There is much debate on this in the presence of only limited empirical research (Bruininks *et al.*, 1980; Felce, 1986).

The philosophy of normalization together with the researched therapeutic advantages and government policies, have enabled community developments for people who are mentally handicapped to become a reality. It is vital, however, to develop a clear picture of who the services are for, and what are the needs of people who have been living in mental handicap institutions for many years.

PEOPLE LIVING IN INSTITUTIONS

Visitors to long-stay mental handicap institutions are likely to encounter people living there who have been admitted for a variety of reasons, arising from social circumstances, physical and/or mental illness.

The emotional and financial demands, inadequate community support services, and inability to accept the handicapped family member can often lead to admission to an institution. This may also follow a bereavement, particularly amongst older people with mental handicaps living with elderly parents (Oswin, 1985) or under the Mental Health Act (Gostin, 1985). The presence of psychiatric symptoms such as irritability, depression or anxiety may precipitate admission (Nosvogel, 1984); the combination of physical, mental handicap and behavioural difficulties may be better dealt with

19

medical, paramedical and educational facilities immediately at hand. Various behavioural problems have been observed as the very reason for institutionalization and failure of community placements (Eyman and Call, 1977).

Of older residents of mental handicap institutions, the circumstances surrounding their admissions may be surprising. Being orphaned, suffering from epilepsy, being illegitimate, having a child out of wedlock or a minor physical disability, such as a squint, being pigeon-toed or particularly small, have been noted by the author to be criteria for admission of older residents (60s upwards) to a long-stay mental handicap institution. This needs to be seen in the context of what was defined as socially aberrant at the time of admission (e.g. illegitimacy), limited medical knowledge (e.g. epilepsy), and inadequate community resources and contacts, then and up till the present to enable a 'normal' life in the community. (For further reading see Wolfensberger, 1975.)

Institutionalization

Numerous writers have pointed to the importance of lack of community contact in the process of institutionalization (Barton, 1956; Goffman, 1961; Sommer and Osmond, 1973). This can result in the 'loss' of friends and relatives, and of the knowledge and skills necessary for social interaction and use of community facilities.

Institutionalization has been described as an 'iatrogenic (physician-induced) disease' (Brody, 1973), manifested in people in long-stay hospitals by depersonalization, dependence, low self-esteem, lack of occupation or fruitful use of time, geographic and social distance from family, friends and cultural milieu, lack of freedom, desexualization and infantilization, crowded conditions and negative, disrespectful or belittling staff attitudes. Residents may exhibit these signs to various degrees and combinations.

By contrast, researchers have noted residents of mental handicap hospitals to have become less socially dependent, and show higher IQs in accordance with their length of stay (Balla, Butterfield and Zigler, 1974; Balla and Zigler, 1975). People with mental handicaps from deprived homes appear to improve in institutions (Zigler and Williams, 1963). Residents have been shown to be more autonomous problem-solvers and have higher language skills than non-institutionalized people with mental handicaps (Yandot and Zigler, 1971)!

The effects of institutionalization are likely to vary in accordance with individual differences and needs. Institutionalized, as against individualized, behaviour may indeed be an asset for survival in the institution (in contrast to the experience of McMurphy in 'One flew over the cuckoo's nest', Kesey 1962) but a handicap to community living. Fortunately, researchers have indicated constructive interventions that may be employed in the process of de-institutionalization and community integration.

FACTORS ENABLING SUCCESSFUL COMMUNITY INTEGRATION AND DE-INSTITUTIONALIZATION

In the last 20 years, there have been many and varied programmes implemented to enable people with mental handicap to move back to the community from long-stay hospitals.

In an overview of research findings by Bruininks *et al.* (1980), the following conclusions were drawn:

1. Community 'success' of the individual is directly related to the quality of training received in the institution, particularly in aspects of personal behaviour on which the individual will be judged in community life, e.g. sexual behaviour, socially acceptable usage of alcohol, grooming, dealing with strangers (Menolascino, 1977);
2. Community support is a vital ingredient for community programmes to be successful, e.g. acceptance by the public of people with mental handicaps as neighbours, employees, and as citizens possessing human and civil rights as well as allowing access to existing services;
3. The planning of the move must be the result of co-ordination, co-operation and consultation, between the institution, community staff, and the client and his/her family, in order to keep everyone informed and to ensure that appropriate community services are organized and accessed for the client. A suggested plan to follow includes: (a) involvement of staff members from the community and institution in order to provide the client (and themselves!) with a feeling that both parties care about the client's needs and desires; (b) a site visit by the client to the new facility; (c) involvement of the client in the preparation of his/her personal affects before the move; (d) involvement of the family in the moving and readjustment process; and (e) the appointment of a

personal advocate for the client to provide advice, support and friendship (Cochran, Sran and Varano 1977);

4. Support and follow-up of the individual once he/she has moved are essential to ensure that he/she has access to the facilities needed in order to survive in the community with a 'reasonable' quality of life;

5. Financial support by governments is likely to be required in order to set up additional services or access existing services to a larger population;

6. Community personnel need to be well trained and versed in a wide variety of skills in order to help individuals 'settle-in'.

Tjosvold and Tjosvold (1983) point to care staff practices which aid both the development and integration of mentally handicapped people into the community – (a) implementation of client-centred care, whereby the functioning of the house/hostel is based around the needs of individuals; (b) involvement of clients in home management issues, such as payment of bills and interpersonal conflicts, through 'house meetings'; (c) enhancing the sense of 'control one one's destiny' by involving the client establishing his/her own 'aims' and 'goals'; and (d) use of peer interaction to help clients learn from and with each other.

Characteristics of individuals have been observed to influence re-integration into the community from long-stay institutions (Crawford, Aiello and Thompson, 1979). Sex, age, IQ and area of pre-admission residence are sometimes predictive of success in family care (Jackson and Butler, 1963). Age has found to correlate positively with successful adaptation to community life and IQ to correlate positively with legal problems (Windle, 1962), which is probably not advantageous to integration in the community.

Variations in staff numbers, style of work and attitudes towards the client, as well as the house layout and organization of the home have been observed by Bjaanes and Butler (1974) to influence community integration. Crawford, Aiello and Thompson (1979) take the view that the system of support available to carers, as well as the client, may be the most important factor in determining whether a person who is mentally handicapped can remain in the community or is sent back to the institution.

INFLUENCE OF GOVERNMENT POLICY ON COMMUNITY PROGRAMMES AND WORKERS

Researchers have indicated factors such as style of work of carers, individual difference of clients, accessibility of community services and follow-up of individuals as influencing the relative ease (or difficulty) with which people with mental handicaps can settle into community life. The ability to get programmes going and have money available is largely dictated by government policy, which may or may not consider the suggestions of researchers, but is likely to be swayed by opportunities for cost effectiveness.

Scandals have also provided an impetus for changes in government policy. For example, the Ely Hospital enquiry in Britain has been said to have precipitated the 1971 White Paper *Better Services for the Mentally Handicapped* (1971) (Donges, 1982; Russell, 1985). Also, the 1980 Committee of Inquiry into the care of children with mental handicaps living at St Nicholas Hospital in Melbourne resulted in the closure of the hospital and rehousing of the children in small groups in the community, with necessary supports (Crossley and McDonald, 1984).

Scandals may provide a catalyst for change, but are no guarantee for continued political commitment for financial support needed in order to ensure a high standard of care. The ability to carry on a job in the face of doubtful funding and/or poor development of community services poses practical problems for workers involved.

PREPARING FOR THE MOVE TO THE COMMUNITY

Moving people from a long-stay institution into the community can be seen as having three distinct phases: assessment, active preparation and community integration. Each stage requires the occupational therapist to perform certain tasks. The assessment of clients prior to a community move will be dealt with in Chapter 3. The remainder of this chapter will examine the tasks that the OT must perform in the active preparation and community integration phases, in addition to preparing the families and community concerned, and working with community support staff.

Active preparation phase

The length and intensity of the work done by the OT in the active preparation phase will depend on the client's disabilities and projected needs in the community. Work done should follow on from the 'results' of the assessment phase (Chapter 3). In general however, the OT should:

1. Inform the community staff as to what he/she sees as the client's abilities and limitations with regard to ADL, kitchen and living skills;
2. Order any equipment, and commence training programmes, given the availability of facilities and time;
3. Locate and introduce the client to any clubs, centres or employment training programmes prior to departure from the institution;
4. Together with care staff, the OT should ensure that the client has opportunities to visit the neighbourhood on several occasions;
5. Visit the new accommodation with the client to check that it is accessible. Any alterations and adaptations must be forwarded to the relevant authority and any work done must be checked (Chapter 5);
6. Any furniture and kitchen equipment must be purchased at this time, and the OT must indicate what particular features are required.

The tasks done by the OT at this stage will be variable and dependant on the individual's needs, as is illustrated in the case study (Appendix 1).

Within the literature, some specific programmes run by OTs at this stage include a social skills/discussion group where feelings about the impending move were aired (McGowen, 1986), and using a training flat in the hospital grounds (Bodenham, 1983).

Some potential difficulties that may hinder the OT at this stage include: (a) absence of suitable facilities to talk to clients privately or to run programmes; (b) difficulty maintaining clients' interest or attention in whatever you are trying to engage him/her in; (c) delays in locating or refurbishing suitable accommodation for the client outside the institution (Halliday and Potts, 1987); (d) no community support staff to work with and hand over to with regard to specific techniques, management; and (e) having to fit in around the client and ward routine, which may be quite rigid.

These are mentioned not to be off putting, rather to acknowledge that preparing clients for the move is a complex task, and that the OT needs to be quite flexible in his/her approach to make sure all the jobs get done.

Community phase

This commences from the time the client leaves the hospital grounds on the way to his/her home. Despite much preparation by the client and care staff, with regard to the new home, location of amenities, etc., it is invariably a busy and stressful time. Researchers have noted that the move may well cause transition shock in the client, a state of being manifested by bodily and psychological reactions to the move (Coffman and Harris, 1980; Gathercole, 1981b; Heller, 1982; Allen, 1989). Suddenly, the individual has to deal with a new set of values, physical and social environment, difficulties that people face whenever they move (Coffman and Harris, 1980).

Extreme responses to resettlement from long-stay hospitals by people with mental handicaps include depression, refusal of food, weight loss and weeping (Gathercole, 1981b), disturbed sleep, gastrointestinal problems and aggressive outbursts (Coffman and Harris, 1980). Kleinberg and Galligan (1983) observed that clients who were severely intellectually impaired showed an increase in antisocial behaviours. Heller (1982) notes that deterioration in physical health and mortality are not uncommon responses to relocation.

Transition shock has been observed to have two distinct phases, firstly, dissatisfaction with the new setting and secondly idealization of the former setting (Coffman and Harris, 1980). It may not appear immediately, with the delay due to the buoying effects of initial optimism, fascination, plus extra attention for new arrivals. The researchers caution, however, that in time, the effort of 'coping' every day takes its toll, and that even people who seem to be managing very well outwardly, both socially and vocationally, may be experiencing extreme stress.

Optimistically, transition shock may be influenced by the amount of preparation the individual has had prior to the move, the individual's personal resources, such as health and social skills, the maintenance of routine, family and friendship ties, and the expectations of the move (Heller, 1982; Allen, 1989). Opportunities for choice and independent decision-making, family involvement in planning the move, and early appointment of care staff helping the person to

25

move may also ease the shock. These findings give some practical leads to those involved in helping people to settle into community life – helping friends to stay in contact, encouraging the client and family to be involved in decision-making, working in with community staff whilst the client is still in the institution, etc.

In between the physical and psychological traumas, there are many tasks for the client and care staff to do. This includes locating medical practitioners, dentists, local amenities, sorting out pensions/ social security or unemployment benefits, setting up the house or just settling the client and his/her possessions in it.

It is very hard to generalize as to what the OT should do at this stage but he/she should, in principal, be following on various actions commenced in the previous stage, in close collaboration with the client and any care staff involved. This may include the implementation of ADL programmes, such as bathing or dressing, kitchen skills, such as tea and sandwich making, or locating and introduction to local leisure facilities and social clubs, etc. Any apparent problems with mobility and safety within the house must be tackled. Aids and appliances ordered and fitted must be checked with the client and carers to ensure correct usage and safety.

It is impossible to anticipate all of the teething problems; needless to say experience has shown them to be more numerous than anticipated. The case study (Appendix 1) illustrates this also.

Having made the move, and with basic OT tasks completed, the therapist should then be in a position to withdraw, and respond to requests for intervention from the client, carers or Individual Programme Planning (IPP) meeting (Chapter 4). In the author's experience, this has included requests for aids, rails, help with structuring and organizing skills training programmes, organizing further adaptation to the home, helping clients to seek employment, ordering wheelchairs, shopping for furniture, and organizing craft materials for staff to run activity groups with clients.

PREPARATION OF RELATIVES AND FRIENDS

The importance of preparing close relatives and friends of people soon to return from mental handicap hospitals to the community cannot be underestimated. Family acceptance and involvement in their relative's move to the community has been observed to be a significant factor in determining successful community placement and employment (Schalock and Lilley, 1986).

Attitudes to de-institutionalization

Just as the diagnosis of mental handicap and institutionalization of the family member will have likely precipitated a 'crisis' for the family, the return of that person to the community is likely to 'trigger off' a reaction (Bartnik, 1981). The decision made years previously to institutionalize the person, perhaps with the encouragement of medical personnel, in the belief that it was 'the right thing to do' is suddenly overturned; community care is seen to be 'better'.

Despite enthusiasm for the concept of community care, Halliday (1987) notes some parental anxieties, given that the parents had already tried to care for their relatives at home but had failed. Concerns related to: (a) the safety of the home, such as the danger of falling downstairs or the risk of injury inflicted by another resident; (b) negative reactions of neighbours; (c) the possibility of the relative 'failing' in the new home, and having to return to the institution; (d) the compatability of staff and residents, and how this could be ensured if somebody left and was replaced; and (e) the success of the home being so dependent on the care staff's approach and attitude. The parents were observed to be ambivalent about the close proximity to their relative and whether they should visit their relative more often. Other parental reactions noticed by this author include fear of invasion of privacy, of having increased responsibility for the relative, and that the relative would not receive appropriate medical attention if required. Researchers have also indicated a preference amongst parents/guardians of people with mental handicaps for their relative to remain in a current placement, be it in an institution or the community (Rudie and Riedl, 1984).

Involving relatives/friends

As research indicates, families should be involved and informed of the process of their relative's impending move. This does not necessarily have to solely be the task of the OT. In many community teams this task is shared and often the hospital staff are involved. Whatever the arrangement it is, there should be clear agreement on the method and timing with regard to presenting relatives with information about he impending move. One way of doing this is to involve the relative in the assessment process (Chapter 3 and Appendix 1), individual plans (Chapter 4), and keeping him/her informed about the move. Evans et al. (1986) noted the valuable contribution

27

of parents of mentally-handicapped adults in planning the Welsh service (All Wales Strategy).

One may well encounter a relative whose views and actions may not to be in the client's best interests. Failing the use of tact, and deployment of the relative's energy into a constructive channel, such as a self-help group, one might consider engaging an advocate (Chapter 8) for the client.

For those clients without nearby relatives or friends, the care staff involved will likely have to work that much harder to create a sense of 'family' for that person. The possibilities of a 'foster' family, befriender or an advocate to enlarge the client's social network should be investigated.

Reactions of relatives/friends post-move

Some of the reactions and concerns of parents after their relatives had moved include: (a) more frequent contact with the relative and care staff; (b) belief that the move had been beneficial to their relative; and (c) reduction in anxieties about the relative living in the community (Halliday, 1987). By contrast they were also concerned that their relative might have an aggressive outburst and put others in the house at risk, a reversal of an earlier fear, and that the staff were overworked and unsupported. Some were unsure about their role in relation to the house, given that their relative had other 'parents'.

Halliday observed that most parents felt an upsurge of guilt within the first year. Seeing their relatives in a home not too dissimilar to their own made parents feel as if they should have been able to cope. This 'guilt' was not always recognized by parents; instead they tended to diffuse their guilt by finding small faults in the house, the staff or in how they ran the house.

These reactions are mentioned by way of illustration, to indicate some of the issues that might be aroused in relatives and friends of clients who have recently moved into the community. It is important to both to recognize these reactions and to put them into context of the relative's experiences. Some of the ways in which the relatives' fears can be channelled constructively have been mentioned.

PREPARATION OF THE COMMUNITY

Like the clients and his/her family, the community at large requires some preparation to receive ex-residents of mental handicap institutions into its midst. 'Community', in this instance, refers to neighbours, shopkeepers, people that the client might come in contact within the course of daily life, or through voluntary and statutory organizations.

Importance of community support

The degree to which ex-residents integrate into community life could be said to be directly proportional to the degree to which the community is prepared. The timing and location of placement appear to depend primarily on the quality of community support than on the characteristics of individuals (Bruininks *et al.*, 1980). Commitment from outside agencies is required, and also agreement to co-ordinate services to the consumers concerned.

Community resistance is often based on uninformed fears regarding the behaviour of people who are mentally handicapped, and that real estate values will be drastically affected by the presence of a group home in the neighbourhood (Lippman, 1976; Bruininks *et al.*, 1980). Berdiansky and Parker (1977), reporting on the establishment of group homes in North Carolina, indicated that the primary objectives voiced by group home neighbours concerned the possibility of danger to their families and sexual deviance. Resistance has also been observed in publications such as *Not on our Block* and statements such as 'Our neighbourhood isn't zoned for it' or 'These grown men with the minds of children will be a menace to our daughters' (Lippman, 1976).

Promoting community support

As well as indicating the influence of community attitudes in the development of community housing and programmes for adults with mental handicap, researchers, fortunately, have been able to identify ways to allay community fears and promotion of a more positive outlook.

Involvement of the community in the planning process appears to be a key way in which positive public attitudes can be fostered and policies made relevant. Lippman (1976) notes the development of a co-operative relationship amongst parent organizations, government officials and the press in the Scandinavian countries, which has enabled the status of mentally handicapped people to be improved in the public's eye through efficient dissemination of information. Evans *et al.* (1986) mention the important contribution made by voluntary organizations and parents, in the planning of All Wales (Mental Handicap Service) Strategy. Bartnik, Jones and Hunter (1981) describe a two-day workshop involving a wide range of personnel and organizations to develop policies and programmes for adults with mental handicaps. As a consequence of the workshop the authors noted: (a) increased understanding of the clients' point of view; (b) differing expectations of the clients and their needs were communicated between the various groups represented; and (c) the indentification of organizational, staff, and client goals with regard to the process of de-institutionalization, which were later adopted by the state mental handicap service as policy. Some practical approaches with regard to informing the community listed by Gathercole (1981a) include meeting local parent and voluntary groups to discuss the processes involved in moving people out of an institution. Key people in the community who can lead local opinion, such as councillors or the community health council (CHC) should be approached, and the information disseminated through meetings, conferences, press, radio and television. Fears and fantasies expressed by the community should be dealt with as they arise; it may be counter-productive to reassure people before their fears are expressed.

Working with community organizations on practical tasks can be helpful in gaining support. It is a concrete way in which therapists and planners can show their appreciation of that organization, as well as learn how it works. That may make it easier to refer clients in the future and gain co-operation of the organization in the re-settlement process.

Informing neighbours

The decision as to whether or not to inform neighbours as to 'who is moving in next door' is indeed difficult. Leyin (1988) describes a variety of approaches to this problem. Informing neighbours may be a means to gain the neighbourhood's co-operation, in the hope that they will befriend the newcomers. Fleming (1984) found that early consultation of local residents led to acceptance of a project housing six people with mental handicaps in their neighbourhood, although the very opposite reaction has also been noted (Lippman 1976; Berdiansky and Parker, 1977). On the other hand, 'normally' people don't inform their neighbours-to-be that they are moving in next door; why should mentally handicapped people be treated differently in this regard? As a general rule, any pressure by neighbours to 'inspect' the house should be resisted, in order to protect the client's privacy. A situation may arise where a client's behaviour may constitute a severe disruption to the neighbourhood. Care staff may have to take drastic action to avoid the house 'being seen' in a negative way.

Importance of interagency co-ordination and co-operation

Much has been said about the importance of interagency co-ordination and co-operation with regard to the delivery of health care services in general, particularly the elderly (Stevenson, 1985; White, 1985). With regard to mental handicap services, the National Development Group (1978) clearly indicated that services in the UK could only develop successfully if the National Health Service and local government services were fully co-ordinated, and education, housing and employment were involved in planning. This is because the presented needs of people with a mental handicap are met by a number of services (Plank, 1979). This view was also supported by the 1981 Report of the Development Group for Services to Mentally Handicapped People in the Guy's District (1981), with the liaison and close co-ordination of services as an important feature to be incorporated in setting up a community services for people with a mental handicap.

One of he most important areas requiring co-ordination is the tie between the community residence and those services which involve the clients on a daily basis, for example, local shops, workshops, day centres and schools (Bruininks et al., 1980). These comments seem obvious, although research based on field work indicates that effective co-ordination between services is hard to achieve in practice (Revans 1975a,b; Baquer, 1976; Heron, 1982;).

The difficulties experienced in co-ordination of services can be related to:

1. Differing management structures and styles between organizations – this was noted to be a problem during the planning of the All Wales Strategy (Evans et al., 1986).

31

2. The number of services that are often involved in order to maintain people in the community, e.g. 'Mary' (Chapter 6), a woman of 65 years with learning difficulties, and a history of depression and agoraphobia, living with her mother of 91 years, received support from:
   (a) the occupational therapist and community support worker who helped her to develop independence skills and maintain a routine;
   (b) a psychiatrist, who had to organize several admissions to a local psychiatric unit;
   (c) a social worker, who organized Mary's finances, day centre placement, and accommodation;
   (d) two home helps who escorted Mary to and from the bus on the days she went to the Activity Therapy Centre (ATC) (Mary's severe agoraphobia made it impossible for her to get to the bus stop alone);
   (e) two volunteers who accompanied Mary to Adult Education classes, near the ATC;
   (f) the council housing department, who was renting the flat to Mary and her mother;
   (g) a GP;
   (h) the mobile library – Mary was a keen reader;
   (i) the home chiropody service.
3. Finding time to liaise with community groups, given the demands of a heavy caseload and other commitments.

Given that many clients having made the move to the community may be in 'transition shock' (Coffman and Harris, 1980; Gathercole, 1981b; Heller, 1982; Allen, 1989), it is not unreasonable to suggest that good interagency co-ordination and co-operation could eliminate potential sources of stress. This is an area which OTs do need to contribute to, in order to minimize overlaps, define the difficult problems and maximize available resources (Bowden, 1985).

Various methods that could be used to achieve better co-ordination between services include: (a) consultation of all relevant organizations during the planning stages (Freedman, 1988a) of a move for a specific client; (b) on-going liaison between agencies after the client moves; and (c) identifying a procedure for review of client care before the client moves, e.g. each agency monitoring the service it provides to the client and/or one agency naming a particular worker to co-ordinate all the relevant services, as in the individual plan system.

Maintaining regular contact with community organizations takes time. The positive outcome is that the agencies feel included and are more likely to be enthusiastic, and could also offer relevant information and expertise to planners. Given the demands of client work and administrative duties, often community practitioners can only liaise with a limited number of agencies. It is quite possible that the community mental handicap team could benefit from having an additional worker whose role would be to liaise with and discover groups or services existing in the locality (Vickerman, 1985), which could uncover valuable resources to aid clients to integrate into the community.

WORKING WITH SUPPORT STAFF TO ACHIEVE OT AIMS

In a staffed housing situation, it is fair to suggest that the people most involved in enabling clients to settle in and adapt to community living are the care staff working in the house or hostel. The care staff carry a lot of responsibility, and often have to make difficult decisions with or for the client. They must know when to call in specialist professionals. The expertise of the care staff becomes more critical as the level of impairment of the client becomes more profound (Eyman and Call, 1977). Surveys of care staff working in the community support a need for additional training, especially for clients with behaviour problems (Bruininks *et al.*, 1980).

Staff play a major role in the creation and maintenance of a high quality of life (McCord, 1981) and their competence is a crucial factor in determining the success or failure of the client to adapt to the community (Bruininks *et al.*, 1980). A major anxiety of parents with regard to the community move of their mentally handicapped children is that the service provided in the community home is proportional to the skills and interest of the staff (Halliday, 1987).

Training of care staff

The view that 'quality of care' (i.e. oriented to the individual) given to people with mental handicaps is dependent in part on staff practices, has been verified by various authors (Klaber, 1969; Balla, 1976; Baroff, 1980; Tjosvold and Tjosvold, 1983). It therefore follows that care staff must receive relevant training in order to fulfil the demands of the job, and maintain high standards of 'care' and support of clients within the home.

Much has been written about the training, the structure and components that community care staff should receive (Kings Fund, 1980; Felce *et al.*, 1982; Allen 1983; Firth, 1983; Mathieson *et al.*, 1983; Ward, 1984; SETHRA, 1987; Averill, Lee and Felce, 1989; Sperlinger, 1989). References are made to the use of procedural guides (Mathieson *et al.*, 1983), use of board games (SETHRA, 1987), block training occurring over a two-week period, and team building (Allen, 1983), prevention of burnout (Firth, 1983), development of assessment and teaching skills (Kings Fund, 1980), learning about the service one is working in and what one's role is (Ward, 1984) and the importance of inservice training (Bruininks *et al.*, 1980; King's Fund, 1980; Allen, 1983; Ward, 1984).

Generally speaking, induction programmes, often placed at the beginning of the individual's employment cover a wide range of subjects, from learning practical tasks such as lifting and transfers, use of incontinence aids, management of epilepsy, to availability and use of resources in the community, and how to use the skills of various professionals such as physiotherapists, speech therapists, OTs and social workers. Often time is spent discussing normalization philosophy and visiting some of the resources in the community.

The content of any training package is likely to vary, depending on the needs of the clients and the skills of the staff. For staff moving from institutional to community work particular care must be exercised in the educational process (Bruininks *et al.*, 1980; Ward, 1984).

OT involvement in care staff training

Within any induction training package, there is a need for OT input. Indeed, it may be the only opportunity the OT has to speak to the staff in detail about the role and skills of the OT, impart some ideas with regard to disability, and say what input he/she can offer to clients and care staff.

The author had several opportunities to be involved in induction programmes for support staff, many of whom had no formal mental handicap training, who were appointed to staff group homes for mentally handicapped adults. The following were included in induction and inservice training programmes:

1. An hour-long discussion/question session incorporated into the induction programmes, covering the following topics:
   (a) the role of the OT in the community team, including general philosophy of OT, use of aids and adaptations, involvement in

housing layout and design, and advisor on household equipment;
(b) difference and overlaps between OT and PT, OT and psychology with regard to skills training;
(c) demonstration of some commonly used household aids (e.g. dressing, bath and kitchen aids), and situations in which they might be used;
(d) working with other OTs in the community or in nearby hospitals;
(e) equipment available from the OT and procedure for requesting and ordering aids;
(f) involvement in the development of leisure and occupational activities and employment opportunities for clients.

On one occasion, the presentation was done in conjunction with the team's PT; this further enabled staff to see the difference between OT and PT roles.

2. A practical session, where participants were 'assigned' various disabilities (e.g. wheelchair bound, blind-folded, hands bandaged) and were requested to prepare and eat a meal. (Most participants were surprised by the difficulties they encountered and felt they had gained some insight as to how physical disabilities can inhibit the performance of everyday tasks).
3. Follow-up sessions organized for staff working with physically handicapped people covered lifting, transfers, and wheelchair management. The staff were encouraged to visit the Disabled Living Foundation, to view the range of aids there and be made aware of some of the devices which can influence independence in daily life.
4. Functional assessments performed by the OT with clients were done in the presence of the care staff. This provided a further opportunity for the OT to explain what she was doing and how various physical difficulties could be overcome.

Other training sessions that could be incorporated in an inservice training programme include:

1. Mobility in the community, where the participant is assigned a disability (such as blindness, or being wheelchair bound) and sent off into the community to complete various tasks such as shopping in a supermarket, or trying on clothes;
2. Use of eating aids;
3. Sensory integration and stimulation programmes; and
4. Seating and positioning.

Additionally, a library of ADL equipment, books and pamphlets could be set up as a resource for the care staff. However, this should be done only when given a regular time commitment by the OT to administer the library and give adequate publicity.

OUTCOME OF COMMUNITY CARE DEVELOPMENTS: PROBLEMS AND SOLUTIONS

'Successful' integration

Factors such as family involvement (Schalock and Lilley, 1986), preparation of the client and community support (Bruininks *et al.*, 1980), care staff practices, attitudes and availability (Bjaanes and Butler, 1974: Tjosvold and Tjosvold, 1983), government support, both ideologically and financially, have been noted to influence the success of community programmes for people with mental handicaps. Atkinson (1988) includes the following:

1. Personal qualities, e.g. motivation, social skills personality;
2. Close friendships, e.g. moving with a friend;
3. Social contact with friends and family maintained; and
4. Having some kind of daytime activity.

Good preparation of client, and on-going support for care staff (Hemming, Lavender and Pill, 1981) contribute to this also. The use of community facilities and staff practices which enable clients to use them (de Kock *et al.*, 1988) are important, as well as the home being located in an area where there are services (McHatton, Collins and Brooks, 1988). Involving clients in leisure activities with the use of volunteers has been demonstrated to be an effective way to aid community integration (Salzberg and Langford, 1981).

Enough time has passed for researchers to report many examples of 'successful integration of people with mental handicaps into community life (McDevitt *et al.*, 1978; Birenbaum and Re, 1979; Hunt and Smith, 1982; Meyers, 1985; Walters, 1985; Johnson and Wallace, 1986; Jones, 1986; Evans *et al.*, 1987). There appears to be some debate as to what constitutes 'successful integration'. Crawford *et al.* (1979) have noted parameters such as length of stay out of the institution, increases in functional and decreases in non-functional behaviours, and parental classification of the client as successful or unsuccessful. With regard to their own survey which investigated outcome of community placement for 85 people with mental handicaps, Schalock and Lilley (1986) noted that if participation in competitive employment was a criterion for success, then only 29% of their sample could be judged as achieving 'success'. If independent living was the criterion, 64% would qualify and if it was becoming a taxpayer, then only 46% of the sample could be identified as successfully habilitated! They suggest that 'success' may merely disguise other problems, such as loneliness, social isolation, or lack of community support, which they observed amongst 'successful' clients who were living independently but were either unemployed or part-time workers. Therefore community programmes involving such clients need to be carefully monitored.

Some potential difficulties

Some of the difficulties that planners of long-term community care for people with mental handicaps should consider, outlined by Way (1985) include:

1. The cost of running several small community units, with well trained staff;
2. The existence of unrealistic expectations of professionals in the community that severely handicapped people will suddenly improve in a new environment;
3. The danger of forming ghettos of people with severe handicaps if concentrated in a special unit;
4. Lack of interest or education of primary care professionals as to the needs of people with mental handicaps;
5. Difficulty of maintaining, supporting and serving dispersed units within a geographical area;
6. The vulnerability of people with mental handicaps in a competitive and assertive society;
7. The 'release' into the community of a small group of people with unrestrained behaviour which could place members of society at risk;
8. Limited opportunities for peer integration, occupation and recreation for handicapped people if they do not easily integrate into normal community activities; and
9. Confusion and disagreement over the venue for treating people with a mild degree of mental handicap who suffer from additional psychiatric illness – in a general psychiatric ward or a specialized unit.

Unfortunately, some of these comments have borne true. The aim here is not to be alarmist but to present some of the difficulties encountered and some possible solutions.

Problems that have emerged

Finance

The reality of ideological support from government for community developments for people with mental handicaps, but with severe financial restraint, is indeed difficult to deal with. The present organization, administration and quantity of money available for 'Care in the Community' policies in the UK has come in for criticism in recent times (Office of Health Economics, 1986; Timmins, 1986). Constant changes in eligibility, and type of benefits pose a tremendous difficulty for care staff helping to organize client monies. Experience has shown that in practice it can be an extremely time-consuming and slow process organizing the benefits for clients moving out of hospital into the community. This highlights the need for early planning and liaison with the local Social Security office.

There is still much debate with regard to the financial efficacy and cost of community versus institutional care of people with mental handicaps (Bruininks et al., 1980; Office of Health Economics, 1986). Davies (1987) provides an excellent study in comparative costs of three models of residential services in the Bristol area. The figures supplied by Toogood et al. (1988) for the costs of a high quality community service for clients with challenging behaviours are indeed steep. However, researches have noted that the cost entailed in caring for this client group are no more in the community then in an institution (Mayeda and Wai, 1975; Felce, 1986) and that centralization of facilities on a single site (e.g. hospital) is not necessarily cost effective (Felce, 1981). Furthermore the NIMROD project in Wales has found that the expenditure required to support lower dependency clients in their own homes or unstaffed housed is well below the hospital figure, although the cost per week is slightly higher for more dependent people in staffed houses (NIMROD, 1983).

The question of finance with regard to community residential services for people with psychological problems has been summarized by Piasecky, Puttinger, and Rutman (1977). Their findings probably have some application to the funding of community housing for people with mental handicaps, and summarize many of the issues hotly debated:

1. Costs for residential services are related to the staff input required for clients;
2. Differences in cost can be attributed to:
   (a) provision of rehabilitation services in-house;
   (b) number and type of staff employed by the programme; and
   (c) the level of supervision given to the clients;
3. Start-up costs are substantial, often equalling the annual cost for operating the facility;
4. Size, in terms of number of clients, has not been found to be a major deterrent of cost;
5. Facilities operated under government auspices report somewhat higher costs than proprietary and non-project facilities;
6. Substantial geographical and urban rural variations were found;
7. The rate of inflation for residential services has matched or exceeded the general inflation rate.

The funding of community programmes is indeed complex; the variance of opinions with regard to the relative costs of hospital verses community accommodation makes it hard to draw any definite conclusions. It is important, however, to note what the issues are, as the organization of monies in any programme can affect staff morale and one's style of working.

Low morale of hospital and community staff

Staff working in mental handicap hospitals that are in the process of closure, face considerable difficulty in trying to maintain good standards of care for clients (Gaze, 1985). Buildings and gardens do not get their usual maintenance. Not knowing the exact date for the closure of the hospital, many experienced staff leave in search of permanent positions elsewhere. Organizing temporary staff can be difficult, putting more pressure on the staff in post and lowering morale. Constant staff changes affect both residents and community workers alike.

Hospital staff who know the client well, may have left so community workers 'lose' what might be vital information about their client. Community workers have to continually negotiate with different staff as they move or are replaced.

Community teams facing these difficulties should consider employing a worker whose job is to liaise with various wards and hospital staff, to keep track of changes, and keep the staff informed of the community developments. This person could also keep close contact with those residents who don't have community care workers involved with them, and to collect important information from staff prior to their departure. Time spent liaising between the hospital and community could enable closer links to develop between the two which could be invaluable to work with residents, due to move.

Bender (1986) states that real ethical dilemmas face every health professional working under the threat of hospital closure, that might force people to leave their jobs. The desirability of returning *all* residents to the community needs to be examined. For example, can the relocation of elderly persons suffering from senile dementia be justified in terms of client benefit? Planners of community services could alleviate the dilemmas in part by ensuring comprehensive planning, which closely examines existing resources and anticipated future needs (Bender, 1986).

Location of the closing hospital

Institutions tend to be built on the edges of cities and towns. The policy of hospital closure must mean a greater distance between the hospital and the area to which the resident is going to move. This must also mean that time will be spent by workers assessing clients' needs and planning the service travelling between the hospital and the designated patch. Travel is time consuming and tiring. It can also limit the number and type of tasks a worker can achieve in a day. It will make bringing the client up to see his/her new neighbourhood a major exercise and perhaps lengthen the process of organizing a client to move. Managers and planners must support workers in overcoming this difficulty by:

1. Establishing an effective transport system for workers between hospital and the community, for example, a volunteer driver or car pool. The cars would need to be accessible to people with physical disabilities and large enough to carry walking aids, such as wheelchair or walking frame;
2. Making available money to reimburse fares and petrol for those who have cars;
3. Giving consideration as to where the workers are based. Should the base be in the patch or at the hospital? Should it be split between the two areas, for example three days hospital based, and two days in the community? In practice, time wasting is reduced if time is regularly split between the two areas. If this is case, then office space will be required at both venues, with someone always available at either office to type, take messages etc.; such costs will need to be budgeted for.

Delays in opening homes

Delays in organizing and providing accommodation for people moving out of mental handicap hospitals may be very demoralizing for clients, families and workers concerned, as illustrated by the following case study.

Halliday and Potts (1987) examined the effects of a 3-year delay, felt by the clients, parents and staff, due to move into two community homes.

The clients became insecure and lost faith in the staff who were breaking promises by not providing the new home they wee talking about. They were not prepared for the change by their parents or the staff as none of them know when it would take place. Parents and staff feared the move would never take place. The parents were concerned that if there were so many problems at this early stage, that there would be more after the move and the direct care staff felt that they had lost their initial enthusiasm. They felt unable to prepare the clients for the move and resented that they had been forced to break their promise to them and that this would not enhance future friendships or trust. The hospital service was also affected by the delays in this project; future plans were postponed and there was a loss of interest both in implementing them and considering new proposals.

Various strategies were employed in order to cope with the delay. The staff involved themselves in training periods, and some continued to work on specific programmes with the clients concerned. Attempts to involve the clients in choosing furniture and fittings for their new homes were thwarted by Health Authority regulations, tendering procedures and staff shortages.

The main cause of the delay stemmed from the bureaucracy involved in identifying and repairing the two council houses offered, to specified standards. The poor communication between direct care staff and planners was also a significant factor contributing to the delay as well as the inexperience in planning community housing. This made it difficult to attempt short-term solutions and hence the way the project was organized. For further illustration of the impact and causes of delays, see Davison and Saxton (1989).

Other issues

Katz (1968) notes that the absence of adequate community support for people with mental handicaps probably contributes to their returning to an institution. Bouras (1986) suggests that the failure to get community programmes for people with mental handicaps off the ground lies with: (a) resistance from national and local government to provide adequate funds and resources; (b) resistance of influential professionals groups to the need of change, because their interests have become fixed on an existing service pattern; (c) the fact that families of people with mental handicaps are afraid of promises to provide new and alternative services and are anxious as to how effective these may be; and (d) the attitude of society as a whole, which overall might still be in favour of segregation of people with mental handicaps and opposed to their full integration into the community.

Strategies dealing with community and family resistance, and the importance of community services have been discussed earlier on in the chapter. Suffice to say, early planning and anticipation of problems should curb some of the difficulties stemming from these sources. The research of existing and past projects may also prove helpful (British Psychological Society, 1984). Transition shock amongst clients who have moved may manifest itself in a variety of ways; specific staff practices have been indicated as to the handling of prevention of such situations (Coffman and Harris, 1980; Gathercole 1981b).

The need for good interagency co-ordination is paramount if resources are to be developed in a constructive, relevant way and duplication avoided. New services may need to be developed and others extended in order to provide people with mental handicaps the same opportunities as others in the community. Services referred to here include respite care, public transport leisure, and recreation (Bruininks *et al.*, 1980).

Careful assessment of the client's abilities and needs, followed by selection and organization of relevant service, is essential, in order to maintain the client in the community. Unfortunately, the situation of the young man as described by Fullerton (1986), who was placed under considerable stress in a community hostel and could not cope, is a reality. (The young man developed paranoid schizophrenia and was admitted to a psychiatric hospital.)

Final remarks

It may appear depressing to the reader to conclude the chapter on a low note of problems emerging from community developments for people with mental handicaps. However, it is as important to acknowledge the difficulties in moving clients out of mental handicap hospitals as it is to be enthusiastic about developing and setting up the service in the first place. Sober consideration of anticipated difficulties in the planning process may prevent their emergence at a later date. Occupational therapists must be aware of the issues no less than any other workers involved in the preparation and movement of people with mental handicaps out of institutions.

Therapists working in their field, can be cheered by the fact that there are examples of good practice, which clearly demonstrate that it is possible for people with mental handicaps to integrate into community life. Some specific strategies have been indicated for OTs working in the field, with regard to clients, their families and future communities, to enable this goal to be achieved.

3

Assessment

The bulk of this chapter will examine the assessment of people with mental handicaps moving from an institution to the community. Many of the assessments mentioned are of use and relevance with clients already living in the community – at home with their families, with friends or independently. They also can be applied across the spectrum from those with mild to profound handicaps.

ASSESSMENT AND PREPARING CLIENTS FOR THE COMMUNITY

The function of assessment of people who have a mental handicap provides a method to: (a) make a differential diagnosis, and/or decide on 'treatment' approach; (b) identify goals and training needed; (c) review progress; (d) make decisions about placement selection or referral; (e) do research; and (f) provide information for planners and administrators (Harvey, 1986). The latter becomes particularly important when plans are being made to resettle people with mental handicaps back into the community from long-stay institutions.

Planners need to be supplied with the facts about what clients need, in order to plan and provide suitable accommodation, a network of health professionals, care staff and volunteers and access community services/facilities (Humphreys, Lowe and Blunden, 1984; Freedman, 1988b). It is essential that this information is passed on early in the process, in order to plan a quality and client-orientated service, and mobilize the necessary funds. It takes time to forge links with community organizations and the process of planning and organizing housing, whether it be refurbishing an old house or seeking a place in an already existing hostel, is very time consuming indeed.

Health services planned and organized in the absence of comprehensive data regarding consumer needs, are more likely to provide an inadequate service to the clients they are trying to serve. Because OTs are trained to consider the needs of people from a very broad perspective, they are in an excellent position to assess the skills, abilities and needs of clients with mental handicaps moving out of long-stay hospitals back into the community.

OT and assessment

There are three distinct phases of work for the OT to enable the movement of clients to the community from long-stay hospitals: the assessment phase, the active preparation phase and the community phase, the latter two having been examined in the last chapter. In the assessment phase, the OT should aim to:

1. Establish what daily living tasks the client can do already;
2. Identify particular physical, social, leisure and occupational needs;
3. Establish some goals for working with the clients;
4. Identify particular housing needs and estimate how these needs might be best met (e.g. hostel, small group home, warden-controlled flat).

In the literature there are interview-based assessments/questionnaires used to gather information about client skills and needs as a part of the planning for a move to the community (e.g. Humphreys, Lowe and Blunden, 1984; Freedman, 1988b). Although taking a very broad approach and gathering information from carers and relatives as well as the client, those approaches do not involve direct observation of the client in performing any tasks noted. A better approach is that of Cassidy *et al.* (1986) based on the STAR profile (Williams, 1982) which involved observing clients in the performance of tasks.

Important in the assessment and gathering of information for planning is the speed by which it can be done and the facilities available for assessment. Cassidy *et al.* (1986) had an assessment house in the institution grounds, and were able to complete their work without the pressure of the institution closing down. Occupational therapists working in community teams rarely have access to a well set up

45

Table 3.1 Format for collection of basic information

	Comments Person A	Comments Person B	Comments Person C	Comments Person D
Basic information				
a. *General health*				
b. *Brief history* - when admitted - under what circumstances				
c. *Important people* - close friends - family links				
d. *How client spends his/her time* e.g. typical day, goes to classes/centres, work				
e. *Additional information from case records*				

assessment area in the institution, and must also work very fast in order to establish what resources clients will need. On this basis, the author used the following assessments to gather information needed as quickly as possible in order to establish clients' support, housing, leisure and occupational needs. They are not standardized, but do provide a global approach, involving observation and gathering information from carers, relatives and case records.

Basic information

This should include:

1. Personal details – name, age, date of birth;
2. Reason for admission to hospital and date this occurred;
3. Brief history within the hospital, number of wards the client has lived in, participation in any day programmes, work, holidays, etc.;
4. General health of client – physical and psychological;
5. How the client spends his/her time – it might be useful to ask the client to describe a typical day;
6. Friendship networks and family links – this particular relevance as to where the client moves to, and with whom. Table 3.1 shows a format that could be used to gather information. Columns have been provided for information to be gathered from the client, nursing/care staff, relatives or friends for comparison. Differences in comments indicate the need for detailed observation and assessment.

ADL assessment

This serves to gather basic information about the client's level of independence in this area and to roughly estimate why skills could be absent – physical handicap, lack of practice, impaired brain function due to damage or disease, etc. It is easier to identify physical barriers to the performance of daily living tasks, and how those problems may be remedied. A basic assessment should give the OT an estimate of the housing and support needs of the client, as well as what ADL skills he/she possesses.

There is a plethora of assessments available that can be used to assess independence in daily living tasks. Wallender, Hubert and Schroeder (1983) describe 29 assessments in great detail, some of which have been particularly designed for use in group homes. Eakin (1989a,b) describes ADL assessments used by occupational therapists, and emphasizes the importance of standardization. The ADL assessment used by the author with clients about to move into the community was not standardized but sufficient to make some early planning decisions and goals. A domestic assessment has been separated off for special consideration.

The ADL assessment may be tackled in several ways:

1. Assessment by observing the client performing tasks in the ward/training area as part of their daily routine, i.e. being present during bathing, dressing, meal times, and general observation of the client. This may be very time consuming and difficult to arrange.
2. Assessment on the ward – this should provide a clear picture of the client's present functioning in the institution. It may not give any indication of the client's *potential* for independence because of the physical limitations of the assessment area.
3. Assessment in an area outside the ward, with appropriate facilities and range of aids and appliances. This may need to take place outside the hospital in the absence of an area that is adequately set up. It should give the OT a clearer idea of what the client's potential is, as against current functioning in the ward.

It is advisable to attempt assessment on the ward first, and then to proceed to use an external facility. The client should be accompanied by someone who knows him/her well, for example a key worker or a relative. It may not be possible or practical to get the client to do exactly what you want – he/she may not want to be active when you want to do the assessment. One should be prepared to use other estimates to gain an idea of a clients level of functioning at a *physical* level. For example, it may be impractical for the OT to arrange to be on the ward to observe the client dressing or bathing. Instead, one could ask the client to take on/off a cardigan/jacket, shoes and socks and perform a few movements, such as placing his hands on his head, shoulders, knees and toes.

As a rule of thumb, if the client can:

- Touch his toes, it is likely that there are no *physical impediments* to him washing his feet or putting on shoes and socks.
- Put his hands on his head, then it is likely that there are no physical restrictions to him washing his back, brush his hair or putting on a jumper.
- Touch his shoulders and knees, then it is likely that there are no physical barriers for the client to wash himself between these two areas.
- Touch his knees and is able to grasp your hand, it is likely that there are no physical impediments to putting on a pair of underpants.

Having to approximate a client's abilities is most undesirable. However, in practice one may not have the time to do more before having to submit, for example, an estimate of how much support a client requires to perform basic daily living tasks. It is better to base such an estimate on minimal but direct observation and assessment rather than on heresay or guesswork.

The OT might also consider doing ADL assessments with a physiotherapist. It may enable the assessment to be done faster, provide a second opinion and promote good working relationships.

The OT should not be disheartened if he/she does not complete the ADL assessment in one visit or session. He/she must be sensitive to the client's concentration span, tolerance of being moved about and having to deal with yet another new face. A suggested format for an ADL assessment is laid out in Table 3.2 with additional columns for information gathered from others working with or who know the client well.

Domestic and Living Skills Assessment

The aim of this assessment is to ascertain if the client has any kitchen skills, and to observe hand function in particular. The

Table 3.2 Format ADL assessment

Client's Name .... Assessor ....
Address .... Date ....
D.O.B. ....
Next of Kin and Address ....

	Assessor's observations	Comments Person A	Comments Person B	Comments Person C

a. *Mobility*
 - walking
 - stairs
 - transfers
  - sitting to standing and vice versa
  - in/out bed
  - in/off toilet
  - in/out bath
 - any mobility aids e.g. wheelchair, frame				

b. *Feet* - type of shoe - any oedema in legs				
c. *Bathing* - wash front, back, hair, feet - any aids used e.g. bath mat, rail				
d. *Toilet* - know when to go - continence - any aids used e.g. rail				
e. *Dressing* - top half of body - bottom half of body - shoes and socks - any aids used - sits on bed/chair to dress - chooses own clothes				
f. *Eating* - feed self - hold cup/drink - any aids used				
g. *Personal hygiene* - clean teeth - brush hair - shave - manage periods				

(contd)

Table 3.2 *contd.*

	Assessor's observations	Comments Person A	Comments Person B	Comments Person C

h. *Other skills*
  - money handling
  - writing letters
  - telling time
  - using telephone
  - public transport
  - other				

i. *Communication skills*
  - initiates conversation
  - no speech
  - responds to questions asked
  - words used
  - any sign systems e.g. Makaton, Rebus				

outcome of this assessment should give the OT an idea of what kind of kitchen appliances and kitchen/household features should be considered as well as what other living skills the client has. A basic assessment should cover the following:

1. Sandwich making
2. Tea making
3. Turning water taps on/off
4. Turning a cooker and oven on/off
5. Opening an oven door
6. Opening the door of the refrigerator
7. Turning light switch on/off
8. Putting an electric appliance into a socket and turning the switch on/off
9. Opening/closing doors using a key
10. Opening a window
11. Bed making
12. Hand washing of clothes

With regard to the ADL and domestic/living skills assessment, the OT must bear in mind that the ability of the client to perform a task is a reflection of the opportunities and exposure the client has had to practice the task. For example, a person may not be able to get in and out of the bath independently because he/she has always been lifted in a hoist as the nurses felt this was the most efficient means of performing the procedure. Or a person may not know how to use a telephone because he/she has never had an opportunity to use one.

Housing and support needs

Based on the ADL and domestic assessments, the OT should be able to estimate what the client's housing and support needs are in terms of:

1. Type of accommodation, e.g. small group home, wheelchair accessible throughout, warden-controlled flat, hostel, nursing home;
2. What people the client might like to live with, e.g. close to or far away from relatives, special friends;
3. Where the client would like to live – particular geographic area, location that enables access to familiar community facilities;
4. The need for particular household features and household appliances; the OT needs to consider the individual needs of the client room by room. These are summarized in the housing checklist (Table 3.3).
5. Support needs of the client, i.e. does the client need 24-hour support for most aspects of daily living or for budgeting, shopping and cooking, or only requires daily visits or could live alone, in warden controlled flat etc.

The case studies of 'Harry' and 'David', a young man with profound mental handicap (Appendix 1), illustrates how the assessments thus far can be used.

Occupational and Leisure needs

These must also be identified early, in order to search for appropriate resources. A suggested formation for the gathering of this information is the Daytime Activities Questionnaire in Appendix 2. It is based on a form designed by the North Southwark CMHT who used it to identify leisure and occupational needs of clients moving back to the community from a long-stay hospital. The use of such a form is likely to produce an *underestimation* of resources needed, given that clients surveyed will likely have had only limited opportunities to develop leisure and occupational interests whilst in the institution.

Table 3.3 Housing check list. Housing features required to maximize independence of client

Client's Name .... OT .... Date ....

Household features	Comments

1. Housing type
   (ground floor/two storey, flat, house)
2. Entrances
   (ramp, threshold flush)
3. Width - doorways
       - passageways
   (900 mm in for wheelchair users)
4. Height - light switches
       door handles
       socket outlets
       window openers
       telephone
5. Type - light switch
       door handle
       window openers
       telephone
       floor coverings
       doors
       door closers
       taps
6. Placement of fire blanket, fire
   extinguisher; height fire alarm
7. Bathroom
   - size
   - bath or shower
   - siting of bath or shower
   - rails/other aids
   - wash basin - cantilevered or other
                  - siting
                  - type
   - flooring
8. Toilet area
   - size
   - rails/other aids
   - siting of toilet bowl
   - wash basin - cantilevered or other
                  - siting
9. Kitchen
   - height of sink, work areas and
     cupboards
   - special selection required for stove,
     refrigerator, washing machine
10. Bedroom
    - easy access to toilet/bathroom
    - size
    - call button
    - special features (e.g. strong joists)

Further comments

However, it has been found to be useful in identifying the number of day centre places required in ATCs and old people's centres, people who would like to work, a range of activities that need to be accessed to clients and how this may be achieved, e.g. use of volunteers, creation of new jobs. The results are detailed in Appendix 2.

For further discussion on the organization and planning of leisure and occupational opportunities, see Chapter 8.

OTHER ASSESSMENT TOOLS

There is a variety of assessment tools which the OT can employ to gather extremely detailed information about a client's ability to perform daily living tasks. These include the Portage Guide to Early Education (Bluma et al., 1976). The Beereweeke Skill Teaching System (Felce *et al.*, 1986) STAR (Williams, 1982), and Learning to Cope (Whelan and Speake, 1979).

They are not so useful if one is attempting to gather basic information quickly for planning purposes. Their main use is in identifying and establishing areas for skill training.

The Beereweeke Skill Training System is particularly helpful in assessment of clients with profound mental handicaps. There may be a need with such clients for detailed assessment of physical handicaps, as in the Paths to Mobility checklist (Presland, 1982). For further discussion on assessment tool for people with a mental handicap see Harvey (1986) and Peck and Chia (1988).

WHERE TO ASSESS

In theory, it is always best to assess a client in his/her usual living environment, in order to obtain relevant information within the context of a daily routine. In practice, this may not be very desirable particularly if: (a) there are distractions in the home, including others interfering, trying to help or sabotage the process; and (b) the place where the client is being assessed does not give a fair picture of his/her skills, as in the case of a hospital ward where, for example, opportunity to assess bathing and dressing skills in privacy are limited, or cooking facilities are absent.

The importance of privacy whilst doing assessments cannot be overemphasized. The community OT may well need alternative venues to assess clients, much as in the OT department of a general hospital or a community health centre. Assessment outside the client's usual environment may be the only way the OT can obtain an objective assessment of skills and needs with privacy.

SUMMARY

Clear assessment of a client's skills and needs facilitates planning of resources needed and identifies the area for the OT to work on with the client. In this chapter a number of assessment tools that can be used with clients, prior to moving to the community from an institution, whilst living in the community, and for clients with wide ranging abilities and disabilities, have been reviewed.

4

Living skills and training

SKILL DEVELOPMENT AND SELECTION

When trying to teach living skills with any client, the OT must decide whether to take a 'developmental' or 'splinter skills' approach, i.e. whether to teach a skill by progressing through the various stages in sequence, or devising a way for the individual to perform the task fairly quickly. For example, if a client has poor grasp and cannot open a door, the OT will have to decide between developing the client's hand skills and building up muscle strength versus finding a mechanical means to open the door, e.g. by installing an electronic door that opens via remote control. In the situation where a person only wears a tracksuit and slip-on shoes, there is a strong case for the therapist teaching the person how to dress/undress with regard to these items only. The skills of doing up buttons or tying laces are not relevant on a practical day-to-day basis (although they are on a developmental scale).

Deciding which approach to take can be difficult at times. Following the developmental continuum is important with children, including those with mental handicap, because of their flexibility and potential for growth. Less support is given for this approach for adults with severe and profound handicaps – splinter skills are advocated here (Lederman, 1984; Brown et al., 1985). However, each client needs to be assessed carefully in this regard – using a developmental approach may be most appropriate with some adult clients.

Factors also important in the selection of skills to be developed with this client group noted by Brown et al. (1985) include:

1. Skills that will enhance the functioning of the individual in a greater number of environments;

55

2. Skills taught are age appropriate, and have the agreement of carers/relatives, so that programmes can be followed through;
3. That skills needed in adulthood are taught early on, so that the individual has more time to practice and perfect the skill;
4. That the individual should participate in deciding which skill to learn first, in order to select skills that have relevance and meaning and will motivate the client;
5. That the skill being developed would enhance the individual's physical well-being and enhance social status;
6. That the skill will enable the individual to have appropriate social contact with non-disabled people in the community;
7. That the individual will be likely to acquire the skill being taught.

It is important that wherever possible:

1. Skills are practiced at a specific time of day (particularly to highlight their relevance, e.g. dressing in the morning), as well as provide consistency; and
2. That new tasks being learned are extensions of those already mastered (Copeland, Ford and Solon, 1976).

Physical disability also affects the ability to master a skill; OTs have a great contribution to make in enabling such clients to master skills with the use of aids and equipment.

TECHNIQUES

The techniques described below all have relevance and are easily applied in the community setting. Some can take place easily in the house (e.g. reinforcement, tactile stimulation) and others might be better suited in the context of a community facility (e.g. puppetry, socialization games). Some thought may need to be given to the particular use of some techniques (e.g. cueing, tactile stimulation) in public places, such as parks, swimming pools and shops.

Environmental influences

In order to enhance learning, the environment in which teaching takes place should be free from distractions. Copeland, Ford and Solon, (1976) suggest that a small room where only the 'tools' needed for training should be used, although this may be hard to achieve in a normal home. Additionally, distractions tend to be very individual (e.g. natural sunlight coming into a room) and require particular vigilance on the part of the therapist in order to identify and eliminate them.

Other factors that can enhance learning and reduce distractions include:

1. The arrangement of furniture in the room – tables and chairs can be arranged to create a 'cosy corner' to work in;
2. Keeping the work surface (e.g. in the kitchen) free of other equipment apart from the items being used;
3. The positioning of the therapist next to the client, to block out visual distractions and enhance a sense of 'closeness' and parti- cipation in the activity: This varies, depending on the task being presented. For example, if in the kitchen, standing next to the client would be appropriate; if teaching dressing skills, it could be more appropriate to stand opposite the client, in order to 'mirror' certain actions for the person to copy;
4. *Some* people find it easier to concentrate, or perform a task, if there is some noise, such as a radio, or if music is playing.

Also important in the enhancement of learning is the elimination of any physical barriers in the environment. This may involve the OT in either adapting the environment or using equipment that will enable the client to overcome any physical barriers that prevent him from performing the task at hand.

Therapist presentation

The manner in which the therapist presents himself/herself when teach- ing, will also influence learning. The following can be very useful in terms of 'engaging' the client and keeping him involved in the activity:

1. Presenting oneself as enthusiastic about a task, feigning it if necessary; if the therapist isn't interested, one can hardly expect the client to be;
2. Planning one's day so that one has the energy to be 'enthusiastic and chatty';
3. Being firm with the client, e.g. if an agreement is made to do cooking, then it must be followed through;

4. Using simple language;
5. If involved in a lengthy task (such as cooking), it can be helpful to discuss other (food) related issues or have a list of other things to talk about with the client whilst working (this works best with more able clients);
6. Limiting the time of the activity – have a rough plan of how long it will take to do certain tasks but also to have a limit;
7. Consider positioning in relation to the client (see Environmental influences, above).

Brudenell (1986) emphasizes the importance of establishing non-verbal communication via eye contact, touching position and gentle voice with profoundly handicapped clients, as a precursor to training.

Copeland, Ford and Solon, (1976) also note the importance of therapist/trainer consistency in the teaching of skills.

Interference in learning

Generally speaking, for clients with behaviours that are interfering with their 'learning', and general participation in an activity, the OT needs to: (a) identify the behaviour; (b) assess its form and occurrence in detail; (c) identify any triggers to such behaviour, and from this (d) identify and eliminate any distractions.

Case example

Nina, was a very active 25 year old, despite the severity of her handicaps. She could not walk, but could crawl very quickly; she had no speech but was very interested in gaining staff attention. She was dependent on staff assistance for dressing, toileting and bathing, although she could eat independently.

Nina came up to the therapy department for an assessment. Within a few minutes she had managed to hit the clients and staff in the room, overturn several pieces of furniture and empty boxes full of puzzles and materials. This was seen in part as an expression of her excitement, but staff learnt that in future visits, they would need to modify the environment considerably by: (a) making sure no other clients were around; (b) only leaving out materials for Nina's session; (c) keeping to a strict time limit for her sessions; and (d) have care staff take Nina back to the ward immediately if her behaviour became violent or destructive.

It may also be useful to identify any likes which can be used as rewards in therapy, or teaching sessions. (In the example above, the reward was being able to come to the therapy department, with the threat of immediate removal if she becomes aggressive.)

Task analysis

Important in the teaching of skills to people with mental handicaps are task analysis and teaching in steps.

Task analysis requires the therapist to 'break down' the task into its component parts in order to construct a teaching programme that presents each part in a logical order that can be achieved by the individual. With more disabled clients, these steps may need to be quite small, in order for the individual to achieve success. For example, the task of drinking involves:

1. Picking up a glass/cup with one or both hands;
2. Lifting the cup to the mouth;
3. Opening mouth and pouring liquid in.

This task can be further broken down to:

1. Putting hand(s) next to cup/glass;
2. Putting hand(s) around cup/glass;
3. Lifting cup/glass towards mouth;
4. Tilting head back;
5. Opening mouth and pouring liquid in.

Having broken the task down into its component parts, the OT can then utilize a number of procedures in order to teach the task. These include behavioural techniques such as chaining, reinforcement, cueing, fading and using equipment.

Behavioural techniques

Of the many behavioural techniques used, the application of chaining, reinforcement and cueing are of particular relevance to the OT.

Chaining Chaining refers to the teaching of skills in a step-by-step process. There are two types of chaining – forward chaining and backward chaining. This refers to the order in which the individual proceeds through the various steps. In the above example (of drinking), if forward chaining was to be used, then the therapist would work with the individual to acquire skills in the order of 1 to 5, concentrating on the next skill once the previous one has been mastered.

If backward chaining was to be used, then the therapist would concentrate on the individual learning the tasks in the reverse order, beginning with skill acquisition at Step 5.

The decision to use forward or backward chaining depends on: (a) the ability of the individual to perform any of the component tasks; and (b) if some parts are easier than others to master.

In general, it is better for the individual to be able to succeed early on in training; therefore, the direction of chaining should take into account what steps the individual can do already, or is more likely to succeed in doing. In the above example, if the person was able to pick up a cup (Steps 1–3), then forward chaining should follow. If the person was able to open his mouth and pour liquid in but could not pick up the cup, then backward chaining should follow.

Dunn and Moorehouse (1980) have found backward chaining to be more suitable for severely and moderately handicapped people, because the individual experiences the reward of completing the task. Copeland, Ford and Solon, (1976) have set out charts for use in teaching ADL using forward or backward chaining. They emphasize the importance of recording the outcome when teaching, in terms of visual reinforcement for the client by means of chart, and as a means for the therapist to evaluate the success of the training programme.

Reinforcement Reinforcers provide a consequence to the individual for a particular behaviour; they are likened to a feedback system (Dunn and Moorehouse, 1980). After a person performs a particular behaviour, he/she receives feedback or a consequence for that behaviour, which will either be pleasant (positive reinforcement) or unpleasant (negative reinforcement or punishment).

Types of reinforcers. Positive reinforcers can be:

1. Social – words, or physical contact – kisses, hugs, squeezes, raise, anything that lets the individual know that his behaviour was approved. These may need to be exaggerated in order to ensure that the person understands that the therapist strongly approves of his behaviour

Table 4.1 Example of a chart used with a female client to provide positive reinforcement and monitoring (items selected were those performed frequently and well by client) ✓ = task completed

Wk beg.	Vacuum-ing	Sweeping	Dusting	Washing dishes	Hand washing	Making tea
Monday						
Tuesday						
Wednesday						
Thursday						
Friday						
Saturday						
Sunday						

2. Tangible – food, water, juice, watching TV, going on an outing – any item or activity which the person enjoys.
3. Generalized – can be traded for either a tangible or social reinforcer. For example, a person may be given a token or a point for performance of a behaviour, and at a specified time, may be able to trade these tokens/points for such things as food, free time, etc. (Dunn and Moorehouse, 1980).

Charts can provide visual reinforcement for task achievement; generally they require the therapist/carer to fill in the chart as tasks are performed although more able clients can fill in their own. Charts also provide the therapist with feedback with regard to the relative success of a programme. Table 4.1 is an example of a chart used with a female client to: (a) monitor domestic activities performed during the week (low levels of activity were an indication of depression), and (b) give the client some visual proof of the tasks achieved. The client filled in the chart fairly reliably; occasionally the OT checked with her mother (with whom she lived) for further confirmation. The therapist reviewed the chart with the client weekly and gave her praise for the tasks achieved.

Negative reinforcers can be:

1. Verbal, and should redirect the individual back to the task at hand, for example, 'Don't hold the knife by the blade, hold it by the handle';

2. Physical – such as spanking – not very appropriate to use with adults, and questionable with children also;
3. Tangible – withdrawal of a pleasurable activity, such as watching TV.

Time-out is often used as a form of punishment/negative reinforcement, when the individual is withdrawn from the activity completely, for example by going to a quiet room for a set period of time (e.g. 2–3 minutes) to 'cool off'. Technically time-out is neither a negative nor a positive reinforcer, although operationally it should probably be considered as a form of punishment (Dunn and Moorehouse, 1980).

Using reinforcers. Reinforcement needs to quickly follow the behaviour demonstrated. Dunn and Moorehouse (1980) note:

1. That a delay of more than two seconds is considered too long a time;
2. With severely handicapped individuals, the more immediate the reinforcer, the more powerful its effect;
3. Immediate reinforcement ensures that the correct behaviour is targeted;
4. Tangible and generalized reinforcers should be delivered in conjunction with social consequences (e.g. praise), to make the reward immediate;
5. Reinforcers need to be obvious, e.g. if praise is to be used, it must be expressed loud enough for the person to hear, or a sign used (e.g. Makaton, Rebus) if the person is non-verbal or has poor hearing.

Reinforcers need to be relevant and have meaning to the individual if they are to be effective. They have to be inherently rewarding and pleasing (if positive), and unpleasant (if negative).

Cueing. A cue is a signal to a person to perform a particular action. Cues used in teaching skills may be:

1. Physical, involving the therapist/teacher putting the client in the right position and helping him/her to perform the task, e.g. in order to encourage a client to put on socks, the therapist may need to:
   (a) Make sure the person is seated;

(b) Place the sock in his hands as appropriate;

(c) Pull the hands holding the sock down to the foot;

(d) Ease the foot into the sock entrance; and

(e) Grab on to the sock (client still holding) in order to draw it up.

2. Sensory, either visual or tactile. Getting the individual to watch whilst a task/movement is performed is an example of a visual cue (e.g. reaching down to one's own foot in order to cue the client to reach his foot in order to put on a sock). Visual cueing requires the therapist to be in clear view of the client, either in front or to his/her side, with no visual distractions. Another kind of visual cue is a marker. For example, markers made of a material that contrasts with a particular garment may be used in dressing to indicate to the client which way a garment should be put on (Goven *et al.*, 1984).

A tactile cue is one which reminds the person to perform a task by using touch, for example, the marker mentioned in dressing above, could also have tactile qualities, such as in the rough side of Velcro. Tapping the hands and foot could serve as a cue to the individual in the process of putting on a sock.

3. Verbal, as in directions to perform a task, e.g. 'Put on your shoes and socks'; verbal cues must be audible to the individual.

All of these cues may be used in the teaching of a particular skill. They can be graded in their use for individuals who need the most direction, from physical, tactile, visual and verbal, with the ultimate aim of no cues being needed.

Fading. Fading is defined as the gradual elimination of reinforcers or cues (Dunn and Moorhouse, 1980). Reinforcers used whenever an individual performs a task should be faded out gradually, for example, from every time the task is completed, to every second, third, fourth time, etc. Exaggerated reinforcers such as food or tokens, should be eliminated before social reinforcers, for example, if food and social praise are to be used as reinforcers for task performance, then food should be eliminated first, only being used every second, third, fourth, time etc.; and then social praise eliminated in the same way, with independent achievement of the task being the natural reinforcer. Cues also should be faded out, if possible, although it may be impossible to eliminate tactile cues for a person with poor vision. Physical cues used in dressing, for example, may be replaced by tactile and visual cues, then verbal, with the ultimate aim of independent task completion.

Equipment

There is a wide range of equipment available that may be used in enabling independence of daily living tasks. The importance of identifying physical restrictions and limitations of clients as against 'intellectual' disability cannot be overemphasized. Particular reference to seating, feeding, dressing, toilets and bathing with regard to equipment will be made later in this chapter.

Pictures and diagrams

Use of pictures and diagrams when teaching skills is particularly useful for clients with deafness. They are another kind of visual cue, and can reinforce the steps to be taken in pictorial form (Figure 4.1).

Picture sequences are a very useful form for recipes for people who can't read (see later). For further reading about pictorial instruction, see Spellman *et al.*, (1978).

Tactile stimulation

Tactile stimulation refers to the stimulation of sensory organs of individuals by touch, sight, smell or sound, in order to facilitate interaction with the environment. Ayres (1972, 1980) has made an enormous contribution with regard to the use of sensory activities in enhancing sensory integration. Many researchers suggest the possibility that people with mental handicaps may require extra amounts of tactile experiences to develop discriminative responses to tactile stimulation (McCracken, 1975).

Goven *et al.* (1984) outline the particular use and tactile stimulation with people with mental handicap, who demonstrate tactile defensiveness or self-abuse. In both cases the introduction of sensory experiences involved:

1. The therapist touching the client (e.g. slow stroking from the top to the bottom of the spine);
2. The involvement of the client in rubbing talcs, creams, fabrics on the skin and the use of games/toys made with fabrics and designed to enhance sensory stimulus (e.g. dominoes textured with sandpaper; incorporation of bells, vibration into pieces of equipment).

Figure 4.1 Pictorial representations of how to do place setting with knife, fork and plate.

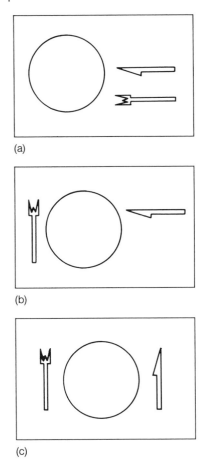

(a)

(b)

(c)

The authors also note the importance of careful assessment in determining the stimuli to be used with each individual. Changes noted amongst children by the authors in response to tactile stimulation include increased tolerance of being touched by others, initiation of social contact by touching (e.g. holding hands or sitting on a person's lap), improved eye contact, interest in peers in the classroom setting and in objects used in teaching. However, reduction in tactile sensitivity was noted to occur slowly – in some cases more than six months – particularly with severely/profoundly mentally handicapped children.

Goven *et al.* (1984) note that tactile stimulation may also be used to:

1. Increase muscle tone in hypotonic muscles;
2. Reduce hyperactivity;
3. Enhance neurological integrates, through visual, auditory, vestibular and proprioceptive perception;
4. Enhance motor planning ability, through improved proprioception.

The main value, however, of using tactile stimulation is to enable the individual to interact with his environment more successfully and to enhance the development of skills. The use of tactile stimulation in teaching activities of daily living has been used successfully by Goven *et al.* (1984). They note that when tactile stimulation is used prior to the teaching of dressing skills, learning seems to take place more rapidly. In this situation, tactile stimulation can be given by firm rubbing or vibration to the particular area concerned. This will be reviewed at length later in the chapter.

Using other media to reinforce skills taught

Occupational therapists often use activities to reinforce the development of gross and fine motor skills and social skills and to enhance a sense of self-esteem and competence. A variety of different media can also be employed with people who are mentally handicapped in order to reinforce the development of independence skills, of which a few examples are mentioned below.

Puppetry and dolls

Puppetry has been used in the teaching of interpersonal skills, sex education and assertion training (Page, 1986). Page noted that normally uncommunicative clients worked very well through a puppet that he/she selected and introduced to the group. Life-like puppets, complete with genitalia were used in a sex education programme, in conjunction with discussion and pictures of males and females, clothed and naked. Page observed that they were useful in assessing sexual understanding. (Astell-Burt (1987) deals with puppetry activities and the teaching of sexuality to people with mental handicaps in some detail.)

Lastly, Page describes an example of using a puppet to develop assertiveness with one client. Performing to the therapist, a client who was very quiet and did not project herself well, was able, via a 'Mr Punch' puppet to tell a story, maintaining the puppet's aggressive character and voice tone, as well as demonstrate how Mr Punch might feel.

Dolls have been used successfully to teach menstrual care techniques, with women with severe and moderate mental handicap (Richman et al., 1986). Through learning to change the pads on dolls, the women were able to generalize this skill to themselves (see later discussion on sexuality).

Role play

In conjunction with modelling and verbal prompting, role play has proved useful in the teaching of grocery shopping to people with severe and moderate mental handicap (Aeschleman, 1984; Wilson, Cuvo and Davis, 1986). It has also been used in the teaching of banking skills, such as opening an account, depositing and withdrawing money, with students who were mildly retarded (Aeschleman and Gedig, 1985). Role play and video could also be used with this client group in the teaching of social skills.

Socialization games

Games that can be used to encourage social skills of adolescents and adults with a mental handicap in a group setting are described by Moxley, Nevil and Edmonson (1980). They have found games effective in holding the interest and attention of participants while they try out a new behavioural repertoire. Incentive to sit in a group, wait turns and try out new activities lies in the laughter, action and recognition of others, generated from the games. There are no winners or losers in the games, and participants can be coached to improve their performance. (This is also the philosophy of 'New Games' (Department of Youth, Sport and Recreation, 1976).) The authors describe games to:

1. Foster physical closeness and distance in an appropriate manner;
2. Helping people to understand themselves and others;
3. Helping others; and
4. Develop social competence.

Games can be selected according to the verbal, physical and cognitive skills of the group. Other useful sources of games include texts by Brandes and Phillips (1977), and Remocker and Storch (1977).

Using groups

Groups can be employed usefully in the teaching of daily living skills and there are advantages to this. Peer group interaction can facilitate learning (Johnson, *et al.*, 1981). Groups are also cost effective and time efficient. Even so, the therapist still needs to have an individual plan or goal for each participant.

The same rules and principles for running groups also apply in the situation where the most handicapped individuals are concerned, i.e. set time, set place, identifying behaviours unacceptable to the group, etc. There needs to be a set criterion for group membership, i.e. only for clients with certain skills and deficiencies. Depending on the nature of the group, it may be desirable to mix the level of abilities. Less able clients can often benefit and learn from those who are more able. For further discussion on group work see Chapter 7.

SPECIFIC ADL AREAS

As a part of planning prior to commencing skill training, or any other activity for that matter, the OT will need to consider:

1. The optimal and most comfortable position for the client to be placed in order to perform the activity, i.e. standing, sitting, lying on his stomach;
2. Equipment required to support the client (e.g. moulded chair, standing frame) in the optimal position for the activity;
3. Equipment needed (e.g. moulded handle on an appliance) in order to perform the task;
4. Whether the task has been broken down into manageable steps for the client;
5. Whether completion of the task will provide a reward for the individual or is an external reward required.

The importance of good positioning to enhance participation and learning is very important with more disabled clients. Seating position has been noted to influence the hand function of people with cerebral palsy (Seeger, Faulkner and Caudrey, 1982). Levitt (1982) suggests that it is important to check for good position and comfort whilst the person is in the chair:

1. That weight is taken equally through both buttocks;
2. That the hips and pelvis are held well back in the seat – straps or a tilt in the seat may be needed;
3. That the back is supported and assess the need for sides on the chair;
4. The height of the chair must be such that both feet are flat on the ground and the table height is correct in relation to the chair;
5. The width of the chair must be such that the person does not slide off the seat; and
6. That the seat and floor are nonslip and the chair is sturdy.

Examples of supportive seating designed for children with poor postural control or cerebral palsy, that could be adapted for use by adults, are described by Finnie (1974), Dawson and Huddleston (1983), Lawson (1983) and Brown (1984). Readers should consult these articles and others listed at the end of the chapter for further details.

Outlines of various techniques and approaches useful in the teaching of ADL are listed below. The areas concentrated on are the ones most important to the acceptance and integration of people with mental handicaps in the community setting. Good references include Whelan and Speake (1979), who list various activities that can be used to reinforce living skills taught, Peck and Chia (1988) and Bender, Valletutti and Bender (1976).

Eating

Given thorough assessment of the individual, the OT may need to tackle training in a number of ways – along developmental lines, looking at positioning, using eating aids, tactile stimulation and cueing.

Programmes along developmental lines

Following a developmental sequence is particularly important for those people who have had no experience in eating independently. Developing pre-eating skills is the first stage. These include swallowing, sucking, mouth opening and closing, tongue control, chewing and biting (Copeland, Ford and Solon, 1976). Various procedures suggested by these authors to develop these skills in children, also have relevance with adults; they include the following:

1. *Swallowing* – can be taught by using a piece of plastic tubing, 16–18 cm in length and 5 cm diameter, dipped in a thin liquid (perhaps of a flavour liked by the individual). The trainer draws 8–9 cm of liquid into the tube, places a finger over the open end, then inserts the tube and releases the liquid onto the back of the person's tongue. If the person is unable to close his mouth, the trainer does this for him. As the person becomes more accustomed to swallowing, the trainer may stroke the person under the throat to facilitate action. Quick icing under the chin can also be used (Lederman, 1984);

2. *Sucking* – the same procedure is used as above, only the tube is placed on the middle of the tongue to stimulate tongue action. Sucking may be promoted by stroking the cheeks, and moving the tube up and down in the person's mouth. A soft bottle (e.g. for tomato sauce) that can be squeezed, with an extended straw inserted in the top may be a useful device; the trainer can force liquid up the straw and towards the mouth. Icypoles or iced lollies will also encourage sucking;

3. *Mouth opening and closure* – mouth opening can be stimulated by touching the lips lightly or using the index finger to apply firm, gentle pressure on the chin, below the lower lip. Pinching the cheeks, stretching the corners of the mouth and using gentle upward pressure under the jaw can facilitate mouth closure. Quick icing around the mouth, and blowing action, such as whistling, picking up pieces of paper by sucking on a straw may also facilitate lip closure (Lederman);

4. *Tongue control* – tongue protraction can be enhanced by using food, such as icypole, that must be licked. Tongue protraction may also be facilitated by pushing on the tongue tip with a tongue depressor, giving it quick stretch; retraction can be stimulated by pulling on the end of the tongue (Lederman);

5. *Chewing* – placing food in the middle of the tongue will indirectly affect chewing. Lips need to remain closed to maintain the chewing action; brushing the lips with the fingers and tapping under the chin will close the mouth. 'Grading' the foods presented, beginning with very soft foods liked by the person, is also important;

6. *Biting* – presentation of food that the person likes encourages this action; gentle pressure on the lower jaw in an upward motion might be required.

Spoon feeding follows on after pre-eating skills. This requires the development of hand – mouth co-ordination, encouraged in six steps:

1. Spreading interesting foods, such as whipped cream or peanut butter, on a table and encouraging the person to dip a finger in and then taste it;
2. Picking up solid, bite-sized pieces of food (e.g. cheese, fruit) from the table; the therapist may need to give physical or verbal assistance;
3. Picking up a spoon from the table – the handle may need to be built up;
4. Lifting the spoon from the table to the mouth;
5. Scooping food with a spoon; using foods that stick easily, such as potato or pumpkin will help here;
6. Bringing the filled spoon to the mouth (Lederman).

Fork feeding and knife usage follow, although Lederman notes that cutting up food is an extremely difficult skill for some clients to master.

Drinking follows the sequence of firstly being a two-handed activity (e.g. using a cup with handles), then one handed. It may be helpful to use a cup with a spout and small amounts of liquid initially.

Eating aids

Some people will never develop all the skills listed, being hindered by physical or cognitive disability, in which case the OT will need to use eating aids to enable the individual to have control over the task. There is a plethora of eating aids available; occasionally, the therapist will need to involve a technician to produce equipment specially designed for use by an individual. Lederman particularly notes the usefulness of the following:

1. Angled spoons or forks may help the individual to reach his/her mouth;
2. Swivel utensils may compensate for the lack of pronation/supination;
3. Light-weight utensils may be used in cases of muscle weakness;

4. Poor grasping ability may be compensated for by built-up handles on utensils or the use of a universal cuff.

Seating and positioning

Correct positioning is important in enabling individuals to develop independence in eating skills, particularly those with a physical disability. Good seating design and the use of 'reflex inhibiting positions' may be helpful.

Steadying the arm and elbow to enable the movement of food from the plate to the mouth is also important. Placing the elbow on the table may steady the action of the arm. Raising the height of the table can reduce the distance that the hand must travel between food and mouth, which may be helpful for people with muscle weakness or restricted movement in the arm.

There may be a use for arm supports (e.g. attached to a wheel chair) or splints, or a weighted cuff, if hand to mouth movements are weak or tremulous.

Tactile stimulation

Tactile sensitivity around the mouth can inhibit the development of eating skills – Goven *et al.* (1984) suggest that tactile stimulation can be usefully employed with such clients. People needing tactile stimulation around the mouth may demonstrate this need by:

1. Excessive fingers-in-the-mouth behaviour;
2. Avoidance of touching around the mouth; or
3. Rejection of anything but bland, smooth food, because of tactile problems inside the mouth.

The authors have found that increasing tactile input around the outside and inside the mouth, and adding refreshing flavours to the mouth can reduce excessive mouthing behaviours. The use of inhibiting procedures, such as neutral warmth or rocking can reduce tactile sensitivity. The vibrator and electric toothbrush have also found to be useful (Farber, 1974).

Cueing

The OT may need to use cues to encourage independent eating. These may be:

1. Physical, such as helping the person to put food on a utensil, or pick up an item of food, and help him take it up to his mouth;
2. Tactile, as in touching the hand and the mouth prior to food being picked up and put in the mouth;
3. Verbal, such as instructions to pick up the food, take it to the mouth, open the mouth, put food in, etc.

The cues need to be graded in their usage, from physical, tactile to verbal (although all may be used initially) and gradually eliminated.

Dressing

The focus for the OT in developing the dressing skills of people with mental handicaps is orientated towards:

1. Using therapeutic activities and techniques to enhance readiness and prerequisite skills for independent dressing;
2. The provision of and training in adaptive aids and techniques;
3. Direct instruction in dressing skills (Lederman).

Prerequisite skills

The following prerequisite skills as listed by Lederman need to be developed in the individual, prior to attempting any dressing training. These include: (a) sitting balance; (b) range of motion (in upper and lower limbs); (c) muscle tone; (d) strength; (e) endurance; (f) grasp; (g) pinch; (h) bilateral co-ordination; (i) visual attention; (j) space, form and figure ground perception; (k) body scheme awareness; (l) motor planning; and (m) memory. Lederman describes in detail in her text activities that the therapist may use in order to develop these skills.

Adaptive aids and special techniques

Regular clothing and dressing techniques are preferable to adaptive methods as they are less expensive, more readily available and provide a greater degree of normalization (Lederman). However, adaptive clothing and aids may also enable independence in dressing. Table 4.2 summarizes various clothes and adaptations to clothing mentioned by Lederman and Goven *et al.* that can be usefully employed with people who have mental handicaps to teach dressing

Table 4.2 Clothing choice and adaptations for specific problems (Lederman, 1984; Goven *et al.*, 1984)

Clothing problem	Adaptation/solution
- putting on socks correctly	Heelless socks; socks with contrasting heels and toes; highlight toe and heel of plain sock with a marker
- difficulty putting on long socks	Shorter socks
- tight fitting socks (e.g. nylon)	Acrylic, orlon, blends (with natural fibres) have greater stretch
Shoes	No bows; slip-on shoes; elastic
- can't do laces	laces (tied up); Velcro fastenings on shoes
Trousers	
- unable to fasten or unfasten	Pants with elastic waist bands (e.g. track suits); use of Velcro fastenings to replace buttons or zips
- discriminate between front and back of trousers	Use of cues to teach front (e.g. place two safety pins, buttons, etc. in front of pants to provide visual and tactile stimuli)
Seams	
- splitting	Stretchy fabrics; reinforce seams and hems; larger size clothing if splitting occurs during dressing/undressing
Buttons/hooks	
- difficulty buttoning and unbuttoning	Polo shirts, skivvys, t-shirts; replace buttons with Velcro discs (sewing buttons to button holes); sew shirt cuff buttons with elasticized threads; button hook
- lining up buttons and button holes	Cues below each buttonhole
- inserting hook into eye (e.g. doing up a bra)	Replace hook and eye with Velcro fastenings (in the case of a bra, front fastening is easier)

skills. Both physical and cognitive disabilities have been considered. For other suggestions regarding clothing design, see Hallenbeck and Behrens (1966) and Moore (1988).

Cues are also useful in helping the individual to orientate clothing correctly. Colour cues can be used in putting on and tying shoe laces (Baldwin, Fredericks and Brodsky, 1984). The big toenail on the left foot can be painted red to correspond with a red dot on the left shoe; half a shoelace can be painted red with the other half remaining white, to provide cues in untying and tying.

Goven *et al.* note the use of cues on clothing in order to indicate the place for the individual to grasp a particular item, in order to pull clothing off or put it on. The authors also note:

1. Cues can be used to indicate the back of a garment, such as a pullover, so that the item is orientated correctly;

2. Cues may vary in size, length, colour and texture, depending on what the individual responds to; the tactile rather than the visual aspect of the cue is more important for people who are more severely handicapped;
3. The size and type of cues may be varied in time, e.g. from a strip of Velcro, down to a safety pin;
4. The use of cues eliminates the need to teach concepts front and back, which are difficult for many people with mental handicap to understand.

The OT may also need to introduce special techniques for people with physical disabilities. Lederman notes the special techniques for hemiparesis and muscle weakness (Trombley and Scott, 1977), and cerebral palsy (Finnie, 1978); where positioning is used to control reflexes that would otherwise make dressing very difficult.

Dressing training

Generally speaking, the teaching of dressing and undressing skills should follow a developmental continuum. Undressing is easier to learn than dressing, so teaching should commence there.

Goven *et al.* particularly note that pyjamas are the easiest garment to teach dressing skills because they are easy to adapt with cues, and cost little, compared to daytime wearing apparel. Pyjamas also tend to be larger than most items of clothing, and take less time to put on/take off when compared with daytime clothes. As with teaching other skills, teaching dressing should follow a step-by-step process, using forward or backward chaining, with appropriate reinforcement, and cues (e.g. physical, verbal) used, as required. Using backward chaining has been noted to be a more effective teaching technique for people with a mental handicap (Lederman). Copeland, Ford and Solon, (1976) have set out sequences in chart form for the teaching of dressing skills.

Tactile stimulation and other activities

In addition to using adapted clothing and cues, Goven, *et al.* have also found tactile stimulation in conjunction with a programme that carefully grades clothing items, to be useful in teaching dressing skills. Tactile stimulation is applied to the palms of the hands, or thumb, if used more in the particular action, prior to the task. For example, the process for learning to put on trousers would entail the following sequence of activities:

75

1. Being able to pull up a thick elastic band (e.g. top of boy's underpants) to the waist. Prior to doing this, with the individual seated:
   (a) Tactile stimulation would be applied to the thumb;
   (b) The trainer would help insert the person's thumbs inside the band at a cue (at the front – to designate front of pants);
   (c) Assist the person in placing both feet through the band, and in pulling up to knees and waist.
   Using this sequence, the individual would then be trained to pull up:
2. An elastic band with a dividing strap, as precursors to trouser legs;
3. Baggy jogging shorts;
4. Elastic waist trousers with cues;
5. Own trousers, with cues, then without.

The whole dressing and undressing process is set out by Goven *et al.* in this way.

Hygiene and personal care

Toileting

Toilet training programmes are of two main types, according to Smith (1979):

1. 'Timing' methods, which involve predicting the time at which an episode of incontinence is likely to take place, and toileting at that time (e.g. Ellis, 1963; Kimbrell *et al.*, 1967; Fewtrell, 1973).
2. Regular potting methods, where the individual is toileted at arbitrarily-set periods of time (e.g. Bettison *et al.*, 1976; Foxx and Azrin, 1973).

The programmes involve collection of base line data, and commonly employ the use of verbal and physical prompting, and equipment, such as pants and toilet alarms (both produce a noise at urination; often toilet alarms can play music – Smith, 1979). The occupational therapist has an important contribution to make here, in terms of programme design, implementation and the mechanical aspects of enabling independence in toiletting. These include the individual's ability:

1. To get to the toilet – the OT may need to identify any barriers, such as a narrow doorway or steps, which impede access for clients using wheelchairs or other walking aids;
2. Manage clothes – dressing and undressing; difficulties experienced may be related to the size of the clothing, elasticity of the material, fastenings being used, hand function and range of movement of joints/limbs involved in executing the task; clothing adaptations and styles useful in overcoming difficulties are listed in Table 4.2;
3. Transfers on and off the toilet – a raised toilet seat or grab rail may be required to deal with problems such as limited range of movement at the hips, muscle weakness in the legs and unsteadiness;
4. Sitting balance on the toilet, or if male, standing balance in front of the toilet bowl – there may be a need for grab rails, for the individual to hold to steady himself/herself; a moulded back support might also be used, if the person is very unsteady sitting on the toilet;
5. To shut the door – a training programme might be needed here, although the person might have difficulty grasping the door handle and pulling it shut; the OT may need to review the type of door handle, and its height from the floor;
6. Wiping the genital/anal area – difficulties here relate to the toilet paper not being within the person's reach, and limited range of movement and strength to perform the task of wiping. A Clos-o-mat toilet provides a warm water action followed by hot air drying of the perineum. A stick with a pincer end (to hold the toilet paper) might also be useful;
7. Flushing the toilet – the individual may find some flushers easier to use than others, e.g. overhead chain pull versus button press. Alternatively, there may be difficulty pressing or pulling these devices, necessitating some kind of adaptation;
8. Washing the hands – lever taps are generally easier than crystal or cross piece tap handles to turn on and off; soap dispensers are sometimes easier to use than ordinary soap; access to the basin, in the home setting, needs to be checked (wheelchair users need basins that are cantilevered in order to reach taps comfortably).

Bathing

The OT particularly has a contribution to make here in terms of enabling physical access to the bath or shower. Commonly getting in and out of the bath is a problem for someone with a physical disability. There is a wide range of aids available from which to choose, including grab rails, non-slip mats, bath boards and seats, and devices to mechanically lower the person into the bath, such as a hoist or Mangar bath seat. Alternatively, difficulty getting in and out of the bath may be related to poor body awareness. It is important for the OT to distinguish this from a physical disability and implement appropriate programmes. Bath inserts, bath frames and hand-held showers (see Appendix 1), are useful when carers have to bath very dependent individuals. Showers will often enable physically disabled clients to be much more independent than a bath. Finnie (1974) provides suggestions for handling people with strong Moro reflex or spasticity. Bathing also provides opportunity for sensory stimulation (Lederman), muscle relaxation and reinforcing body awareness.

Other areas that the OT may need to attend to in relation to bathing include dressing and undressing, transfers in/out of the bath or shower, and handling soap – using a soap mitt can be effective at times.

Personal Hygiene

Teaching personal hygiene, including oral hygiene, nose blowing, hand care, hair care, make-up and deodorant use, is often shared by caretakers, teachers and therapists. The OT can add relevant expertise in terms of adapting some of the equipment used. For example:

1. Oral care – toothbrush handles may need to be enlarged and electric toothbrushes are useful for individuals with poor motor skills (Lederman).
2. Hand care – an emery board can be adapted for one-handed use by slipping it into a wooden dowel with a suction base, and sticking it on a table; this eliminates the need to use scissors.
3. Hair care – long-handled combs/brushes, can be used by people with limited range of movement in the arm; built-up brush handles or selection of a brush with a fat handle can help those with poor grasp.

A group setting can be a good venue to teach grooming skills (Lederman). By learning various tasks and doing them in a group setting, individuals can receive immediate feedback from their peers – this is particularly important in impressing a socially acceptable standard of hygiene.

It can also lend itself to encourage socialization between group members, as well as be a basis for outings (e.g. to the hairdresser/ barber, beauty culture schools).

Use of electric or battery-operated shavers is recommended for use with males who have a mental handicap. The task can be approached firstly by dividing the face into regions: (a) left cheek, (b) right cheek, (c) chin, and (d) upper lip. Shaving must consistently proceed through the regions in the same order each time. By a process of backward chaining and using physical, verbal and tactile prompts, the therapist can encourage the individual to perform the task.

In some situations, the OT may become involved in teaching menstrual care. Research defining specific techniques to teach menstrual care to women who are mentally handicapped is scarce and fails to detail the techniques used (Richman *et al.*, 1986). These authors describe a programme where subjects were taught menstrual care through simulating menstruation with a doll and the subjects themselves. Using a forward chaining process, the authors were able to train the subjects in identifying the menses, and taking appropriate action (changing sanitary pads; disposing of used pad, etc.).

Cooking

Teaching cooking requires the grading of activities to be taught in terms of: (a) the processes involved; (b) the equipment used, and (c) the length of time the task takes to complete. For example, learning to make toast comes before making a sandwich or making a cake.

The OT may need to experiment in finding suitable appliances/ equipment, or adapting what is there already. This is particularly the case with the oven and cooker (Chapter 5). There is a vast range of household aids available for kitchen use, which may be of relevance to some clients. For further discussion on useful kitchen aids and techniques see Conacher (1986).

Recipes may be adapted into a pictorial, step-by-step form. Many recipes have been adapted into pictorial form in an excellent book by Hargreaves (1986). See also a general discussion on the use of pictorial instruction by Spellman *et al.* (1978).

If teaching cooking in groups, shared mealtimes are an excellent venue to develop social skills, particularly with people with severe mental handicaps (Williams, Tyson and Keleher, 1989).

Social skills

There are many definitions of what is meant by 'social skills', although Christoff and Kelly (1983) have been able to define 'social skilfulness' as the 'effectiveness of the behaviour in social interactions (involving) the co-ordination of appropriate verbal and non-verbal responses' (p. 184). Social skills training generally includes conversation skills, listening to others, assertion training and personal presentation. Training programmes have been developed and used for some time with psychiatric patients (Lindsay, 1986).

The move towards integration of people with mental handicaps into the community highlights the need to ensure clients have the opportunity to develop the social skills needed. In a review of current literature, Christoff and Kelly have noted that:

1. Social functioning is a good predictor of interpersonal, vocational and independent living adjustment, amongst people with mild and moderate mental handicap; and
2. That people are more likely to be rejected by others on the basis of inadequate social behaviours rather than mental handicap.

It is safe to assume, therefore that training to improve the social functioning of those clients who have poor social skills, will enhance community acceptance and integration. This has become an important focus for trainers, carers and therapists, given the move towards integration in the community. Conversation skills refers to the ability of the individual to initiate and maintain informal conversations with others (Kelly, 1982). Researchers have suggested that the ability to converse in a 'co-operative' manner facilitates social acceptance of people with mental handicap (Christoff and Kelly, 1983).

Christoff and Kelly note nine programmes which have been successful in developing the conversation skills of people with a mental handicap. Common components in these programmes include:

1. Asking questions of others;
2. Making appropriate self-disclosing statements;
3. Complimenting and acknowledging others;
4. Giving others time to talk.;
5. Making and maintaining eye contact; and
6. Linking body language with verbal content.

What the authors note particularly is the lack of programmes which aim to address the teaching of appropriate conversational topics.

Specific programmes

Many conversational skills programmes involve the use of role play, rehearsal, modelling, video and audio/cassette tapes. Bradlyn *et al.* (1983) describe a successful programme based on that of Kelly (1982), using a combination of techniques in a group setting. The topics being presented to the group of five teenagers were:

1. How to ask appropriate questions and making self-disclosing statements (8 sessions);
2. Making reinforcing/acknowledging comments to others (7 sessions); and
3. Talking about topics of interest to others (9 sessions).

In the 20-minute training sessions, the skill was modelled by the therapist(s) for five minutes after which group members practiced the skill with each other or the therapist. During this time, group members received praise and any corrective feedback from the therapist(s) or others in the group.

As a means to assess how individuals were using their newly-acquired skill, participants were randomly paired after sessions and required to talk for eight minutes whilst being recorded.

They were further required to repeat this procedure with a non-handicapped person. Bradlyn *et al.* (1983) found this method to be very successful in developing conversation skills amongst teenagers with severe to moderate mental handicap.

A programme designed to develop verbal responses to questions or statements amongst people with mild and moderate handicaps is described by Matson and Senatore (1981). The groups consisted of discussions relevant to group members activities in the sheltered workshop where they worked, and covered topics such as specific work tasks, workshop conditions and relationships with workshop staff. Through group discussion, the leader encouraged appropriate responses from other group members to comments made.

Bates (1980) describes a programme for people with mild and moderate handicaps used to develop the following skills:

1. Introduction and small talk;
2. Asking for help;
3. Differing from others, and
4. Handling criticism.

Bates defined 16 situations commonly experienced by participants at 'work', home and in the community. Within group meetings, he worked with clients to develop skills 1 to 4 as appropriate to these settings. Sessions consisted of the two group leaders modelling the situation and appropriate responses, which was followed by group members rehearsing their own responses at least 2–3 times, with one of the group leaders. Other group members watched, and were asked to give the 'performer' feedback. To assist them to give feedback, as well as reinforce the important components of the behaviour, cue cards were distributed, which referred to a different feature of the communication, e.g. eye contact, facial expression, voice volume.

A board game, based on the commercially-available table game 'Sorry' (Parker Brothers), has also been used to teach social skills (Foxx, McMorrow and Schloss, 1983). The skills focused on in the game were compliments, social interaction, politeness, criticism, social confrontation, questions and answers. In order to move forward, the individual had to provide an appropriate social response according to a card picked up.

There are many kits available with video cassettes and/or activities listed that deal with the teaching of social skills. Therapists might find the following particularly useful:

1. The Catch project social skills kit (Sheppard, Pollock and Rayment, 1983), which consists of 6 video cassettes, 9 sound cassettes, an instructor's manual and 19 picture cards;
2. A text by Bender, Valletutti and Bender (1976) which describes activities and approaches in a step-by-step manner;
3. Kelly's (1982) text, which provides clear guidelines for setting up social skills training.

For other descriptions of social skills groups, see also communication and social awareness groups (Chapter 7).

Sex education

The occupational therapist may become involved in the teaching of sex education. Particular points to note in running programmes include:

1. The use of language that is understood best by clients; this may mean the use of slang words, rather than those that are anatomically correct;

2. Asking parents/guardians if they are happy for their son/daughter to be involved in such a programme; this should include providing an overview of the programme, number of sessions, contents, etc.;
3. Using very clear visual aids, such as slides, photographs, films or models of the human body, samples of contraceptive devices, tampons, sanitary pads, etc.;
4. The person running the programme must feel comfortable about talking about sexuality and be up to date on information.

For further information, see the further reading list at the end of the chapter.

Community skills

Public transport training

Public transport training requires the following skills:

1. Recognition of bus/vehicle stop;
2. Recognition of correct bus/vehicle;
3. Paying the fare;
4. Knowing when to get off, and signalling this to the driver as appropriate.

Recognition of numbers (e.g. number of the bus) and extensive money-handling skills are not essential. Individuals unsure if they are on the right bus can be trained to check this with the conductor/other passengers by asking (e.g. 'Is this the bus to Kew?'). For the person who finds organizing the correct money for the fare difficult, he/she can be trained to always use a specific coin or note.

There appear to be two approaches to transport training:

1. On site on a bus, in the community (e.g. Marholin *et al.*, 1979); and
2. In a formal classroom setting (e.g. Neef, Iwata and Page, 1978).

In situ training involves the teaching of bus/train riding skills in a step-by-step approach, with one trainer usually accompanying two or three clients at most (Marholin *et al.*, 1979).

There appears to be some value in teaching in a small group, particularly as the trainer withdraws and there is more demand for the clients to 'perform' – the clients at least have each other to turn to. However, if the expectation is that the client will be travelling alone on a particular route, group training may be contraindicated. The classroom method of teaching, as described by Neef *et al.* involved the use of:

1. A cardboard model, 81.3 x 101.6 cm, simulating four square city blocks and containing cardboard buildings, trees, people, traffic lights, bus stop sign and toy buses; a 7 cm rubber doll with movable arms was used for manipulation by the subjects;
2. A simulated bus, with a coin meter, eight chairs, designations for front and back of the bus and doors and cord to pull; slides were projected onto the front wall in front of the chairs, designated as the front windows, and shown sequenced locations along a city bus route, taken through the front window of a bus on its actual route.

In the study, subjects firstly gained mastery with the doll and cardboard model, then role-played out the desired behaviours with a trainer on the simulated bus.

There is some debate as to which approach is the more effective method of teaching, although Neef *et al.* find both are as effective, with the classroom method being a less expensive way to teach. The classroom method probably has much to commend it when large numbers of people are concerned, and a general skill of public transport training is being taught. However, if teaching a specific route, the on-site method is more relevant and practical for the individual.

Associated with public transport training are road crossing skills. Components of road crossing include:

1. Walking safely along a pavement or on the road, facing oncoming traffic if there is no pavement;
2. Choosing a safe place to cross;
3. Stopping at the kerb or edge of the road;
4. Looking and listening for traffic;
5. Crossing the road when there is no traffic near; and
6. Crossing the road well away from parked vehicles (Taylor and Robinson, 1979).

Again, both *in situ* (Yeaton and Bailey, 1979) and classroom role play and modelling (Page, Iwata and Neef, 1976) are described.

Taylor and Robinson lay out a neat step-by-step programme that teaches road crossing skills using physical and verbal prompts.

Telephone skills

Before proceeding with teaching telephone skills, it is important to eliminate any physical problems which may impede access to or use of the telephone. This might include:

1. The height of the telephone – if too high, it might be difficult for receiver and dial to be reached, or to get a clear view of the numbers on the dial;
2. Dial type – some people find the conventional dial more difficult to use than push button and vice versa;
3. Inability to dial and hold receiver at the same time, e.g. if only have use of one hand – a stand beside the telephone to clip the receiver in might be useful, or, alternatively, a mobile telephone;
4. Poor hearing – unable to hear the telephone ring or hear through the receiver – amplifiers are available, and some people rig a light system whereby the light flashes when the telephone rings.

There are many and varied appliances available to deal with some of these problems. With regard to teaching dialing, Leff (1974) describes some useful aids. These include:

1. Use of discs, placed over the telephone dial
   (a) a disc with 10 different colours, with numbers imposed;
   (b) a disc with 10 different colours, no numbers; and
   (c) 10 colours, for use with push button telephones – there may also be a use for a disc with numbers and colours for button telephones like (a);
2. Telephone numbers written down on a strip of card, with the picture and name of the person being called, followed by the number and appropriate colours (same as dial);
3. A card holder, which allows the picture of the person to be visible, but only one number to be seen at a time.

Using these aids, involves: (a) selection of the most suitable disc type; (b) selection of number to be taught – written on cardboard strip and (c) placing strip in holder and dialing one number at a time, using the colour cues on the strip to match that over the dial. Leff found that with these aids, 91 out of 100 children with a mental handicap, previously unable to dial were able to do so independently.

Similarly, Risley and Cuvo (1980) used pictures to teach emergency telephone numbers. The appropriate telephone numbers were written down next to pictures demonstrating certain situations (e.g. kitchen on fire). Individuals were taught to link certain events with a specific number, using the picture as a cue. This could be adapted further with the use of colour cues for telephone numbers and dial.

For teaching telephone answering, the use of role play, role modelling, practice and reinforcement were suggested by Ballard *et al.* (1987). These authors describe individual programmes to teach this skill, although the group setting is probably also relevant, particularly for role play and feedback.

Shopping and money handling

Shopping lists 'written' in the form of pictures of items are often sufficient prompt to remind clients what they want to purchase (Sarber *et al.*, 1983). Purchasing skills, involving the selection and payment of items, have been taught using role play in a 'mock' shop in the classroom setting (Aeschleman and Schladenhaufen, 1984) and modelling of the desired behaviour by a trainer, in the shop setting (Matson, 1981).

Composing shopping lists is often taught in conjunction with menu planning. Reitz (1984) taught clients to eat and plan more nutritious meals by increasing intake of milk products, fruit and vegetables. This included:

1. Providing subjects with information about food groups;
2. Getting subjects to list what they ate on a daily basis, and paying them 25 cents for each completed card; and
3. Getting subjects to mark off what they had eaten in terms of specific food groups, giving verbal praise when they included milk, fruit and vegetable groups.

A formal classroom setting where clients 'practiced' listing balanced meals, using a series of slides noting particular food items and colour coded for food groups which slotted into a board, divided up into three daily meals, is described by Sarber and Cuvo (1983). A similar procedure is also noted by Wilson, Cuvo and Davis (1986).

Money handling is ultimately connected with shopping. Training programmes can range from teaching an individual to buy specific item(s), e.g. pay for a bus fare or buy a packet of cigarettes, which requires the recognition and use of one coin or note, and collecting any change, to shopping within a budget (Wilson, Cuvo and Davis, 1986) and developing banking skills (Aeschleman and Gedig, 1985).

Developing money-handling skills, however basic, not only can generate satisfaction on the part of the individual, but projects a more positive image to others in the community. Bender, Valletutti and Bender (1976) list various exercises trainers can use to develop money-handling skills with clients.

INDIVIDUAL PLANS

Attention to the needs of the individual, construction of a meaningful life style and organization of appropriate services is the cornerstone of normalization philosophy. The mechanism for facilitating this is through the establishment of Individual Programme Planning (IPP). The main aims of the IPP meeting is to:

1. Help clients and their families express their needs with dignity and obtain, in a co-ordinated fashion, the services needed to meet these needs, and
2. Bring the relevant practitioners and people important to the client together to agree on roles, task, etc. and therefore avoid duplication (Humphreys and Blunden, 1987).

The structure, form and frequency of IPP meetings varies, although components of planning generally include: (a) assessment of individual needs; (b) specification of those needs in behavioural objectives; (c) identification of skills to be taught or actions taken and by whom; and (d) a time scale for completion or review of tasks.

Generally, the client's skills and needs are viewed in terms of self-care, domestic and community skills, leisure, occupation, housing and future needs. Particular training needs are often identified at IPP meetings.

The broad outlook of IPP is commensurate with the OT approach, of looking at clients and their disabilities from a global perspective. Often referrals for OT intervention are made through IPP meetings. Sometimes OTs are involved directly in the chairing or planning of the meeting, if he/she is the identified key worker for a client. The references listed at the end of the chapter describe in considerable detail the structure, running and format of IPP meetings, and organizational setting-up of such a system.

FURTHER READING

ADL

Candish, E. (1984) A feeding workshop for the mentally handicapped. *British Journal of Occupational Therapy*, **47**(3), 79–80.

Carr, J. (1980) *Helping your Handicapped Child: A Step-by-step Guide to Everyday Problems*, Penguin, London.

Dunlap, G., Keogel, R.L. and Koegel, L.K. (1984) Continuity of treatment: toilet training in multiple community settings. *Journal of the Associations for Persons with Severe Handicaps*, **9**(2), 134–41.

Hallas, C.H., Frazer, W.I. and MacGillary, R.C. (1982) *The Care and Training of the Mentally Handicapped*, 7th edn, Wright PSG, Bristol.

Johnson, M. and W. Werner, R.A. (1980) *A Step by Step Learning Guide for Retarded Infants and Children*, Constable, London.

Smith, P.S., Britton, P.G., Johnson, M. and Thomas, D.A. (1975) Problems involved in toilet-training profoundly mentally handicapped adults. *Behaviour Research and Therapy*, **13**, 301–7.

Behavioural Techniques

Kazdin, A.E. (1980) *Behaviour Modification in Applied Settings*, Dorsey, Homewood, Illinois.

Norris, D. (1982) Behavioural approaches to care, in *Profound Mental Handicap* (ed. D. Norris), Costello Educational, Tunbridge Wells.

Perkins, E.A., Taylor P.D. and Capie, A.C.M. (1983) *Helping the Retarded*, British Institute of Mental Handicap, Kidderminster.

Thompson, T. and Grabowski, J. (eds) (1977) *Behaviour Modification of the Mentally Retarded*, 2nd edn, Oxford University Press, New York.

Yule, W. and Carr, J. (eds) (1980) *Behaviour Modification for the Mentally Handicapped*, Croom Helm, London.

Individual Programme Plans

Blunden, R. (1980) *Individual Plans for Mentally Handicapped People: a Draft Procedural Guide*, Mental Handicap in Wales – Applied Research Unit, Cardiff.

Houts, P.S. and Scott, R.A. (1978) *Planning for Client Growth*, University of Pennsylvania, Pittsburg.

Jenkins, J., Felce, D., Togood, S. *et al.* (1988) *Individual Programme Planning: A mechanism for developing plans to meet the specific needs of individuals with mental handicaps*, BIMH, Kidderminster.

Mansell, J., Felce, D., Jenkins, J. *et al.* (1987) *Developing Staffed Housing for People with Mental Handicaps*, Costello Educational, Tunbridge Wells.

Throne, J.M. (1977) Unified programming procedures for the mentally retarded. *Mental Retardation,* **15**(1), 14–17.

Mobility, Seating and Positioning

Bobath, B. (1978) *Adult Hemiplegia: Evaluation and Treatment*, William Heinemann Medical, London.

Bobath, I.C. (1980) *A Neurophysiological Basis for the Treatment of Cerebral Palsy*, London Spastics International Medical/William Heinemann, London.

Brown, S. (1984) An evaluation of chair bases for use on carpet by children with cerebral palsy. *Australian Occupational Therapy Journal* **31** (4), 152–55.

Chia, S.H. (1985) The Bobath approach and its application in OT for children with cerebral palsy. *British Journal of Occupational Therapy* **48** (1), 4–7.

Folkerd, P. and Andrews, J. (1987) Equipment review: the use of colour coding to aid wheelchair management. *British Journal of Occupational Therapy* **50** (2), 52.

Macreill, M., Roser, R.M. and Clarke, E. (1985) Equipment review: the Rutherford kneeling frame. *British Journal of Occupational Therapy,* **48** (1), 19.

Meyers, J. and Massue, B. (1987) *Wheelchairs and their use – a Guide to choosing a Wheelchair*. RADAR, London.

Mulcahy, C.M. (1986) An approach to the assessment of sitting ability for the prescription of seating. *British Journal of Occupational Therapy,* **49** (11), 367–8.

Mulcahy, C.M. and Pountney, T.E. (1987) Equipment review: ramped cushion. *British Journal of Occupational Therapy,* **50** (3), 97.

Presland, J.L. (1982) *Paths to Mobility in Special Care*, British Institute of Mental Handicap, Kidderminster.

Stewart, P.C. and McQuilton, G. (1987) Straddle seating for the cerebral palsied child. *British Journal of Occupational Therapy* **50** (4), 136–8.

Taylor, R.H. (1972) *An approach to designing for the handicapped. Community Health,* **3** (4), 162–6.

Wilson, B. (1980) The development of seating for posturally handicapped children. *Action Magazine*, ISSN 0309 2650, p. 25–8.

Sex Education

Craft, M. and Craft, A. (1977) *Health and Sex Education for the Mentally Handicapped* (Kit: 1 audio cassette (23 min.), 15 colour slides; covers rationale and method.

Craft, M. and Craft, A. (1982) *Sex and the Mentally Handicapped: a Guide for Parents and Carers*, Revised edition, Routledge and Kegan Paul, London.

Kempton, W. (1975) *A Teacher's Guide to Sex Education for People with Learning Disabilities*, Duxburg Press, North Scituate, Massachusetts.

Kempton, W. and Forman, R. (1976) *Guidelines for Training in Sexuality and the Mentally Handicapped.* Planned Parenthood Association, Philadelphia, Pennsylvania.

McCarthy, W. and Fegan, L. (1984) *Sex Education and the Intellectually Handicapped*, Addis Health Science Press, Sydney.

5

Housing

Many references have been made in Chapter 2 with regard to people with mental handicaps living in ordinary housing in the community. There are no special design requirements needed in housing for this client group, unless clients have physical or visual handicaps, which can be dealt with as for other disabled people.

The development of housing schemes does become more complex when specific clients have not been identified for projects, or if one is having to consider future and changing needs of clients. The social needs of clients need to be considered, as do the practicalities of group living situations where the tenants are not necessarily living or functioning as a 'family' group. For these reasons, this chapter has been included. In addition to the above, reference will be made to the selection of fittings, such as ironmongery and kitchen furniture, and working with architects. Case studies and descriptions of housing projects have been included to illustrate some of the difficulties encountered.

Issues relating to the funding of projects have not been dealt with in detail, given variations between countries and regular changes in legislation although some general comments will be made. Furthermore, readers should refer to the reference lists at the end of the chapter for further information about housing in general, and housing projects for mentally handicapped people in particular.

THE ROLE OF THE OT IN HOUSING

The following tasks should be undertaken by any OTs involved in housing in general, and particularly in the housing of people with mental handicaps.

1. Assessment of the client's physical, social, community and support needs, in order to identify suitably located housing that is physically accessible throughout with opportunities for socialization and privacy, as the individual requires (see the case study on 'Harry', pp.105–8, 219–29 for further illustration).
2. Assessment of properties: (a) for development into community houses, and (b) suitability of properties already developed, for example, to see if a sheltered housing scheme or old people's home meets client's needs.
3. Liaison with the architect, if a house is to be refurbished or a major adaptation implemented. This requires the OT to read and check plans, ensuring that passageways are wide enough, sufficient space is allowed for fittings, particularly in kitchen and bathrooms, etc. It may be useful to use 'cut outs' of a wheelchair, bath and toilet to 'check' the plans (Figure 5.1). Architects do vary in their expertise and knowledge of design needs of disabled people. A description of the client and his needs, or if future tenants are unknown, the presentation of some design guidelines to the architect should give a clear indication of what features should be incorporated into the house design or adaptation. Particular points that the OT should note are summarized in Table 5.1. The OT should do a site visit with the architect and client to further clarify any special features required. This should be done room by room, in accordance with the previous housing needs assessment (Chapter 3). At the completion of work done, a further site visit is required to check that there are no problems.
4. Where major kitchen or household items such as cooker, refrigerator, washing machine or dryer are being purchased, the OT should assist the client (and any care staff) in selecting the most suitable appliance in accordance with the client's physical needs.
5. Where it exists, the OT should be involved in the housing management committee (see later in chapter).

For further descriptions on the role of the OT in housing see Dudman and Shaw (1987) and Potton (1980).

CLIENT NEEDS AND HOUSING DESIGN

The type of housing recommended for any client must cater for his/her physical, social and community needs. This is even more

Figure 5.1 Outlines of fittings and furniture drawn to scale 1:50

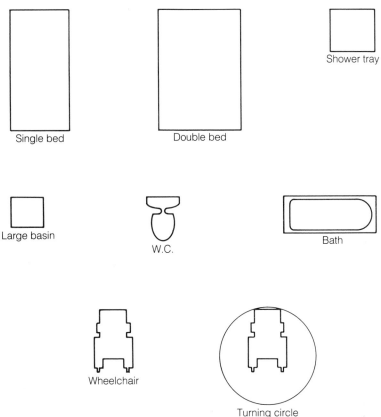

complex if housing is being planned for a large number of people. If the community housing is to be an on-going resource for clients and cater for the future needs of present and potential clients, the design of the house must be flexible enough to cater for severely disabled people also.

Designing for physical needs of clients

It is not an uncommon experience of OTs involved in housing planning, to not know specifically who the client(s) is and what are his/her needs. This has certainly been the experience of OTs working in housing developments for adults with mental handicaps, who need

Table 5.1 Items for OTs to include in design guidelines for architects, assuming clients with mobility problems and ground floor housing

Item	Feature	Comments
1. Bathroom and WC	Layout and space	Cater for users of wheelchairs and walking aids
	Bath or shower	Build in drainage so that bath can be replaced with a shower if required
	Bath	Largest standard length and 0.5 m rim height
	Toilet	Placed adjacent to a wall so that a rail can be attached; space sufficient in front of toilet bowl to enable transfers
	Wash basin	Cantilevered
	Taps	Separate hot and cold; lever taps
2. Kitchen	Work surfaces	Different heights for standing and sitting; pull-out boards useful; worktop to either side of oven
	Plumbing	Flexible hose so that sink height can be adjusted
	Oven, stove, refrigerator	Select with client; consider location to maximize circulation space
	Sink	Install two if more than three-person household
3. Circulation	Passageways and doorsets	Minimum 0.9 m width
	External doors	Near flush threshold
	Ramps	Maximum 1:12 gradient for independent wheelchair use with non-slip surface
4. Other items	Socket outlets	0.5 m above floor
	Window openers, telephone, light switches, door handles	Low enough so that person in a wheelchair can reach
	Door handles	Level handle easier to use
	Storage	Allow space for wheelchair or walking aids
	Floor coverings	Slip resistant in bathroom and kitchen; heavy duty carpet elsewhere; no mats
	Fire precautions	Accessible to tenants; aesthetic
	Joists	Strengthened in bath/bedroom ceilings in case hoist needed
5. Special aids e.g. rail, hoist		Not to be installed before site visit with client and OT

housing in the community. This has meant that the design must be extremely flexible and be able to accommodate the needs of severely disabled people if the housing is to remain a useful future resource. This is particularly the case with any planned ground floor accommodation, although some flexibility, particularly in kitchens and bathrooms, will be required by more physically able clients too. For example, people with Down's syndrome tend to be well below the 'average' for normal height (Heaton-Ward and Willey, 1984), and it is likely that kitchens built with fittings at standard height would be too high for them to use.

Choice of electrical appliances

Particular care needs to be taken with regard to the choice of electrical appliances in the house. It cannot be assumed that all wheelchair users need to have kitchens with split level ovens. This emphasizes: (a) the importance of careful assessment of several products by the OT with the client; and (b) the need for flexible design in the kitchen. Goods referred to here include major appliances such as cooker, washing machine, clothes dryer, refrigerator and television. When selecting goods particular attention must be paid to:

1. Type and arrangement of controls. There is often a variety of gas and electric appliances that one can select, depending on the needs of the client. Controls at the front of an appliance are easier to reach. A guide next to the control, particularly on hotplates can be very useful (Figure 5.2). Push button controls are also useful and easy to use.
2. Safety features. Some hotplate surfaces have a cover that can be pulled down when cooking is finished. Some gas cookers will only release gas when the ignition switch is pushed. Electric cookers, if with elements that glow, are an obvious signal to users that the appliance is switched on. On the other hand, elements take time to cool, when not appearing obviously 'on'. Gas may be easier to control although there are risks if it is accidently turned on but not lit.
3. Height of controls and handles. These must be within the client's reach, particularly for wheelchair users trying to get food out of an oven or refrigerator.
4. Design of control panel. The control panel, particularly on washing machines and dryers, can be confusing with many knobs, buttons and writing to deal with. It is important to assess if the panel can be simplified, for example by colour coding, or covering up of certain buttons.

Figure 5.2 Dots next to control knobs indicate relevant knobs to activate hotplates.

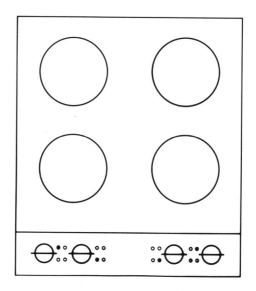

Designing for social needs of clients

The housing must also provide opportunities for privacy and socialization. Designing for the client's privacy is clearly enabled by each person having their own bedroom, and establishing 'rules' as to who can come into the room and when. Creation of 'social' space requires a very large kitchen, with a sitting area, or separate kitchen and lounge. The absence of this extra space was the failure in the accommodation where 'Harry' lived (see Appendix 1 and case study later in this chapter).

A lot of space is required especially when a person with aggressive or demanding behaviour is being accommodated. Other people living in the house may well need to get out of the person's way, if he/she is in an aggressive mood. In this situation there may be a need for two sitting rooms, unless the client concerned has a very large bedroom of their own and can be contained there.

Catering for community needs

If clients are to be encouraged to utilize local services and shops, houses must be located within walking distance of them. Housing not within reach of these services should be rejected. Planners must consider the location of housing also to enable contact with relatives and friends, bearing in mind the observation of Dalgleish (1986) that distance is a determinant of frequency of family contact, particularly if relatives are elderly.

Particular design features to note

1. *Bathrooms and toilets*. It is essential to include a toilet in the bathroom, particularly if clients are incontinent or are wheelchair dependent. In houses where there are more than three people, two bathrooms are needed. Where three or more clients share, two toilets are required, preferably one in the bathroom and a separate WC. This extra space and facilities are required particularly where clients need assistance from care staff or if independence skills in bathing, toiletry, grooming, etc. are to be developed.
2. *Kitchens*. The flexibility of kitchen fittings has already been noted. Additionally, the room must be large enough to cater for the occasions when the clients eat a meal together, with the inclusion, at times of staff, friends or relatives. In practice, kitchens need to be quite large if there is to be adequate space for staff to teach clients to cook. A minimum size of 120 sq ft for houses where six clients live, supported by staff, is recommended by NIMROD (1985).

    In houses where there are five or more clients, two sets of hot plates, one gas and one electric, will probably be needed but only one oven. Refrigerators need to be large (approximately 400 litres storage room) also, particularly when clients are not cooking meals together. Heginbotham (1980, 1981) also notes the importance of having: (a) sufficient storage cupboards, particularly if people are buying their food separately; and (b) an additional kitchenette, away from the main kitchen, in houses where six or more people live, where tea, coffee, small snacks can be made.
3. *Utilities room*. A separate utilities room is needed if the kitchen is to remain useful as a venue for socializing, in addition to

cooking. There is nothing more intrusive than the noise of a washing machine or dryer.

On-site laundry facilities are essential: (a) if someone is incontinent; (b) to cope with the laundry generated by clients and staff, particularly if fresh sheets are to be provided for the latter on a daily basis; and (c) to save money and time being spent at a launderette (Heginbotham, 1981). The utilities room should not be located next to or above a bedroom or lounge area to avoid intrusion of unwanted noise.

4. *Bedrooms.* The minimum size for single and double bedrooms recommended by Heginbotham (1981) are 10 and 15 m^2, respectively. Bedrooms accommodating people with wheelchairs may need to be larger depending on the client's abilities, and any equipment needed. Heginbotham (1981) also notes that clients will need: (a) plenty of storage space in their room, and (b) a lockable bedroom door, to ensure privacy and security of their goods. If staffed accommodation is being organized, staff will need their own bedroom and chance for privacy. Quite likely there will be some paper work for them to do so a desk should also be included, in addition to bed, cupboards, etc. When staff do not have their own space and sleep on the loungeroom couch, the space of others in the house is encroached upon and there is a danger that 'office work' papers, etc. are scattered about.

5. *Fire precautions.* Any fire precaution features to be included must be considered before people move in and refurbishment completed. Clients should know how to use any firefighting equipment, which should be accessible and light enough for them to use (Heginbotham 1981b).

6. *Telephones.* The decision whether to install an ordinary telephone or a pay 'phone requires thought. The inclusion of pay telephones eliminates the difficulty of having to divide up the bill equally and staff could be reimbursed for calls made with regard to their work. However, the processes required for staff to be reimbursed may be tedious and impractical (McCord, 1981) and outgoing calls cannot be made when the machine is full. A regular petty cash float in the appropriate change could resolve the former.

These difficulties need to be balanced against those encountered with an ordinary phone: (a) how will rental and bills be paid? (b) should a client who can't use a phone have to pay a proportion of the bills? (c) should clients pay for calls made on their behalf? and (d) how will calls made by staff that are work related be paid? These questions require resolution prior to anyone moving into the house. Other considerations include the location of the telephone in a part of the house which ensures privacy. It must be positioned at such a height to enable small or wheelchair-bound people to use it.

7. *Other features*. Additional fittings and features considered by Heginbotham (1981) include:

(a) Gardens – need to be not too demanding to keep tidy, and appropriate tools purchased before the house is occupied. Although a good teaching resource and opportunity for exercise, in practice staff often have to do a lot of the work. Gardens need to be accessible to physically disabled people, also;

(b) Carpets – must be of good quality as they get a lot of wear and tear between clients and staff;

(c) Skirtings – tend to get kicked, and with the trend to narrower skirting, walls get kicked too – higher skirtings are useful;

(d) TV aerials – need to be placed in clients' rooms as well as in communal areas (Heginbotham notes that as clients become less institutionalized, they prefer to have their own TVs and watch them in privacy);

(e) Storage –needs to be plentiful;

(f) Central heating – allows bills to be divided up evenly, and reduces fire risks and costs of clients burning heaters in their own rooms;

(g) Insurance and burglary prevention – both need to be organized prior to clients moving in.

Housing people with special needs

People with profound handicaps or behaviour problems can be accommodated in ordinary housing. This has been supported by Cummings *et al.* (1989), who were able to maintain 26 people with challenging behaviours in ordinary houses (n = 19) and flats (n = 16). Thought needs to be given particularly to the size of the house and fittings/furnishings used. For people with behaviour problems, the spaciousness of the accommodation is significant if other clients and staff are to be able to get out of the way during an outburst. It may be advisable to have two lounge rooms in a house for four people in this situation. It is difficult to assess what people's space needs will be, although observing the client in his present situation will provide some guidelines.

Case example:

Sam, aged 35 years, had no physical problems and was very strong. He had no speech, used no sign systems, and would hit people who came too close to him. Opportunities to go out from the locked ward he lived in for the past 5 years were few, and he received no occupational therapy due to staff shortages. The community OT was asked to assess if any special features would be needed in the house that he was to move to.

As a result of discussions with the nursing staff and her own observations of Sam, the OT was able to establish that: (a) Sam liked to have his own space to sit in the ward; (b) he liked being outside in all weather and would often take himself out without prompting; and (c) he spent his time moving between his seat, the garden, the passageway to his bedroom (where he would often pace up and down) and the table where he ate his meals or played with some 'toys'. Given these observations, the OT estimated that Sam would need accommodation that had a garden and a large lounge (about 30 m^2), in addition to kitchen and dining areas, or with two lounges (20 m^2 each).

Fittings and furnishings need to be sturdy and of good quality to cater for heavy use, without looking ugly and institutional. Policies with regard to their replacement, if destroyed wilfully by tenants, need to be established prior to people moving in. There is a good case for tenants having to contribute financially for the repair or replacement of items they damage. The use of toughened glass or glass which turns to powder when broken is worth considering for clients who have a history of putting their fists through windows. Good soundproofing is also important. Cummings *et al.* (1989) required circuit breakers to be installed in one instance.

House grouping

Housing people with severe disabilities and behaviour problems together can be very difficult for staff and clients if a good standard of care is to be maintained (Keene and James, 1986). It is better for all to 'mix' the degree of abilities and disabilities, although this requires more able people to cope with some fairly extreme behaviours. It is particularly important to 'test' this well in advance of the move for all clients, e.g. by sharing time, doing activities together. Carpenter and Axfon (1989) describe the use of a short term residential cottage on the hospital grounds.

Other features to note

For those people with sensory defects, Goldsmith (1984) suggests that the following may need to be considered for the home: (a) an amplified doorbell or visual indicator; (b) an induction loop (i.e. a wire run around a room or house and connected to an electrical appliance, such as a TV. This sets up a magnetic field such that a person wearing a hearing aid with a special pick-up coil can hear the TV without increasing the volume), and (c) good lighting, colour contrasting on corners to highlight hazards, sliding doors and gas cookers.

Features noted by Norris (1982) that could be incorporated in day centres include rooms of regular shape, variations in height and texture of ceilings and floors, use of dimmer switches, brightly painted rooms and colour contrast on doorways and a variety of features in gardens. It is not unreasonable to suggest that some of these features could also be incorporated in housing being developed for profoundly handicapped people.

HOUSING OPTIONS

A wide variety of housing options in the community for people with mental handicaps have been noted by several authors.

1. Staffed group houses, where 3–5 people share a house with 24-hour staff support (Bruininks *et al.*, 1980; Gathercole, 1981a; Towell, 1985; Paterson, 1986) with staff having their own bedrooms to sleep in, rather than being 'waking' night staff. Clients receive assistance and training in daily living skills, seeking of employment, other occupational and recreational pursuits, and integrating into the community in general.
2. A hostel, where clients (approximate numbers are from 6 to 20 people) can receive support from staff in many aspects of daily living and independence skills are developed (Meyers, 1985; Paterson, 1986). There are many variations in management style and organization, ranging from clients pitching in with household tasks, to staff performing all domestic activities. Commonly, hostels are empty by day, as clients are either working, at day centres or involved in some other kind of community activity.
3. Unstaffed group homes, where 3–5 people share a house and receive support from a community worker(s) several times a

week, most commonly to help with budgeting or in time of crisis. (Bruininks *et al*, 1980; Gathercole, 1981a; Towell, 1985). Clients living in this kind of accommodation have many independence skills, including housekeeping, use of public transport and organized daytime and leisure activities.

4. Co-residential homes, where one or more clients share a house/flat with non-handicapped peer(s) who offer support in lieu of rent (Bruininks *et al.*, 1980; Towell, 1985). Co-residents must have acquired considerable daily living skills, and desire living in a shared co-operative group environment. Clients requiring emotional support and encouragement in a group living situation, or who need a positive 'role' model may benefit from such a system. Common problems in this kind of housing include the co-resident taking on the role of a 'staff' member. This may be avoided by the client receiving regular support from the community agency(ies) outside the home, and the availability of support in crisis situations. The co-resident and client should be clear about what the arrangement entails, for how long it is to take place and what are the arrangements for termination of the contract. Even given this, the client may well feel let down or upset if/when the co-resident moves.

5. Nursing and rest homes, which may be appropriate for elderly people with mental handicaps (Paterson, 1986). Paterson notes that elderly non-mentally handicapped people tend to accept elderly mentally handicapped people more readily than any other adult group in society. In this setting, clients receive the same services as others in the home.

6. Sheltered housing, where clients living in small groups or on their own, manage their affairs independently, but can call on support at any time from a nearby warden (Bruininks *et al.*, 1980; Gathercole, 1981a; Walters, 1985; Paterson, 1986). The homes are usually adjacent to each other, and residents often form a mini-society and tend to assist each other. Paterson notes that such housing schemes may create mini-ghettos of handicapped people. If well supervized, however, people living in such schemes can have a full exposure to the benefits of society. Often, however, social work or community worker support is required for the scheme to succeed (Walters, 1985; Paterson, 1986).

7. Boarding houses or lodgings, where private home owners rent rooms to one or more clients, often providing food and personal services (such as laundry and transportation) for an additional

fee (Bruininks *et al.*, 1980; King's Fund, 1980; Paterson, 1986). Clients living in this kind of accommodation exhibit a level of independence similar to those living in unstaffed or sheltered housing. Caution must be exercised with this kind of placement due to the variability that exists in the location, supervision, and quality of accommodation. The establishment of a local landlord and client matching service may be a means to ensure suitable placement, and monitoring of the provisions available.

8. Fostering, where families are paid for caring for a mentally handicapped person. This has been used successfully with children (Bruininks *et al.*, 1980; Gathercole, 1981a; Paterson, 1986), although authors suggest that there is great potential for such schemes for adults. There needs to be careful selection and preparation of client and family, and a system of on-going community support available (Gathercole, 1981a). Difficulties encountered by foster parents include: (a) lack of community acceptance of the client because he/she is handicapped; (b) lack of supportive programmes with regard to daycare, leisure or workshops; (c) lack of medical and dental care; (d) problems with the supervizing agency; (e) problems with the natural parents; (f) intensive supervision demands and lack of freetime, and (g) neglect of other family members (Bruininks *et al.*, 1980).

9. Special care units, for groups of 4–6 individuals, to assess and implement programmes for severely disturbed clients.

The setting up of community housing to cater for the range of disabilities ranging from the most profound to mild mental handicap must include a 'facility' where the needs of people with behaviour problems, and/or psychiatric difficulties may be dealt with, particularly given the closure of 'more secure' facilities, found in mental handicap and mental illness hospitals (Chapter 6). There may be a need for a detailed assessment of a programme to be developed for a client away from the group house, opportunities for short-term care may be required, in the situation where staff and their residents need a 'break' from a very behaviourally-demanding client.

Theoretically, in normalization terms, people with mental handicaps who have psychiatric difficulties should use mainstream psychiatric services. Whilst a most laudable idea, in practice this can be difficult to achieve, given increased pressure on psychiatric beds, because of the reduction in number and associated community developments (e.g. in the USA and UK). While not wishing to see separate services away from the mainstream being set up for people with mental handicap and psychiatric illness, planners may have no option but to do so, in order to ensure that clients at least have access to such a service.

Such accommodation should be very homelike, like staffed housing, but with a higher complement of staff to work with the clients concerned (Bruininks *et al.*, 1980). These authors suggest that placement in such a facility should not be considered permanent, i.e. no longer than one year. However, it may transpire that a client does require such structure and support in his living environment, if he is to develop any skills, or just be maintained at his present level of health and abilities. If advocating a policy that clients should receive services to meet their needs, then it might be the case where they have to continue to live in a very structured environment, as described above.

Housing sources

Houses used in community developments have been noted to come from a variety of sources:

1. Public sector housing, provided by local government (King's Fund, 1980; Gathercole, 1981a; Durrant, 1985);
2. Private sector housing (King's Fund, 1980);
3. Housing organized by voluntary sector and professional housing groups, such as housing associations (King's Fund, 1980; Gathercole, 1981a; Walters, 1985);
4. Housing owned by the State (Hunt and Smith, 1982; Jones, 1986).
5. Housing organized by two or more organizations together (Booth *et al.*, 1989).

There are advantages and disadvantages with each of these sources and the ultimate choice is likely to be governed by finances and speed at which houses must be developed.

Choice of housing

The type of housing recommended for clients will depend on a number of factors: (a) the OT's assessment of the client's physical and social needs; (b) the client's wishes; (c) the relatives' wishes; (d) desired location; (e) cost of types of housing; (f) any district policies or directives towards a certain kind of housing; (g) availability of housing, and (h) speed at which housing must be developed.

The final decision depends on the result of the site visit, particularly if the client has any physical disabilities, and whether the client is able to relate to others already in the house or moving in at the same time.

It is suggested that a range of housing, as listed previously, should be developed to cater for clients' needs and abilities. Experience has shown that two-person flats require the clients to be able to get on extremely well in order to negotiate household tasks and differences of opinion. This may be particularly difficult for people who have lived in an institution for many years, where personal clashes could be diffused by staff or the presence of other residents. It is not recommended for clients moving from institutions to live in a two-person flat as their first choice, unless they are extremely close or that any other living arrangement would prove detrimental and is well illustrated in the following case study.

Case study

Pictured in Figure 5.3 is the ground floor flat that 'Harry' (Appendix 1) and 'Joey' lived in.

A plan of the top floor flat, also designed for two clients, with staff sleep-in support (also available to residents in the ground floor flat), is included. The flat was refurbished by Hummingbird Housing Association (now incorporated into Hyde and Southbank Housing Association) and let to four clients through the Southwark Mental Handicap Consortium.

It was clear from assessment that both men needed to live in ground floor housing; Harry had a mild right hemiplegia, and Joey had cerebral palsy, although could walk quite independently. He needed to be pushed in a wheelchair for long distances.

The men spent a lot of time together during the 9–12 months prior to the move, and they seemed to get on well. A couple of months after the move, however, their relationship deteriorated dramatically, to the stage where they no longer shared meals or talked to each other.

Harry became very impatient and aggressive to both Joey and the support staff. He complained of feeling isolated, bored and that he had no one to talk to. The only space he felt he had in the house was his room, and that the kitchen was too small to sit in if there were more than two people there. Joey, meanwhile, had retreated to his room.

Figure 5.3 (a), (b) Used by two tenants, with one room for staff to sleep in; 908.5 sq ft. (c) The flat where Joey and Harry lived. L/D was used as B2; 534 sq. ft. (With thanks to Peter Mishcon and Associates (Architects) and Hyde and Southbank Housing Association.)

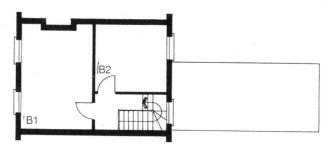

(a) Second

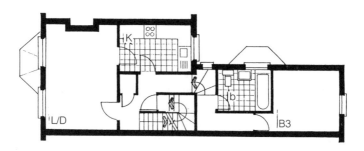

(b) First

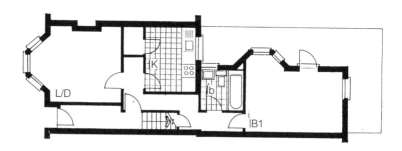

(c) Ground

The support staff found the space in the flat restricting also. Whilst trying to help Harry cope with his frustrations, they found that the only 'neutral' place they could talk to him, if the privacy of his bedroom was to be protected, was the kitchen. This was clearly unsuitable as Joey frequently made himself cups of tea and did a lot of cooking.

The flat did not fully cater for the mens' needs:

1. There was no social space in the flat, with the exception of the kitchen, which was very small. Staff felt it was inappropriate to carry out programmes solely in client's bedrooms, yet at the same time found the kitchen physically cramped and lacked privacy, unless one of the men was out;
2. The usefulness of the kitchen as a social space was negated as soon as the washing machine was turned on;
3. Both men were becoming socially isolated as they kept to their rooms; although Harry could climb the stairs to visit the flat above, Joey could not always do this;
4. Joey occasionally had severe spasms which prevented him from walking even short distances, including going to the bathroom independently.

Not all these problems could be resolved. The only way the social space could be increased was if the two men shared a bedroom, allowing the front bedroom to become a sitting room. Clearly, this was no option, as the two men desperately wanted their own bedrooms, which they had furnished and decorated in their own way. Alternatively, one of the men could move.

An application was made for Harry to move to a larger household with 5 or 6 people, in the hope that this would be more fulfilling for him socially and reduce his feelings of isolation. Hopefully, another tenant would be more compatible for Joey. In the meantime, various tactics focussing on Harry's behaviour were devised by staff in order to maintain the status quo (Appendix 1).

Nothing could be done to change the impact of the noisy washing machine or the narrow doorways and steps which prevented wheelchair manoeuvre to the bathroom from Joey's room. In emergencies when he could not walk to the bathroom, he did use a bottle, and could also have had a commode chair in his room. Even so, this was not a desirable situation, and the severity of Joey's cramps were unknown until after the move. Had the OT been aware of this, a wheelchair-accessible property would have been recommended for him.

This property was successful in creating ground floor accommodation for two people with mild physical handicaps. However, the experience of Joey and Harry has indicated that clients living in such accommodation need to be either: (a) extremely independent and able to cope with bed-sit type living situation or (b) to get on extremely well and be prepared to share a room.

Alternatively, the house could have worked well as a group home, providing accommodation for one person with a mild disability on the ground floor. (This would have required location of a kitchen/ sitting area on the ground floor between the front room and the present kitchen, with the bathroom and the back bedroom as they are. The rooms upstairs could have remained as they were, with the kitchen being replaced by a utility room/kitchenette.) The location of the kitchen on the ground floor would have encouraged contact with the disabled person downstairs, although he/she may not have been able to utilize the laundry facilities upstairs. Such a plan would have meant sacrificing a ground floor bedroom space, but would have created a very congenial environment for 4 people to live in.

INVOLVEMENT OF CLIENTS IN HOUSE PREPARATION

Clients have a vital contribution to make in the preparation of their own home. Whilst not being able to participate in the details of building and design, they should be involved, whenever possible, in choice of bedroom, decorations, curtains and household contents. This provides an opportunity for clients to make a contribution, instead of being 'helpless', and reinforces the reality of the pending move.

However, the experiences of Halliday and Potts (1987) would suggest that this may be hard to achieve. They found their efforts to involve clients in the purchase of their own furniture thwarted by Health Authority regulations, tendering procedures and staff shortages. This indicates the importance of planning specific procedures for purchase of furniture that allow for clients to participate in the process.

In the case of clients who are profoundly handicapped and are unable to actively participate in the process, care staff will have to make the choice for the client, given careful assessment of his/her needs. This may include estimating what colours the client likes, sensitivity to noise, as well as his/her physical and social needs, etc.

MAINTAINING STANDARDS IN HOUSING DEVELOPMENTS

Specified standards with regard to the quality of housing, furnishing and overall service provision to clients in staffed or warden-assisted housing must be set to ensure clients receive a good service. These need to be clarified prior to anyone moving in.

Living environment

The setting of standards in the house should refer to the quality and quantity of: (a) furniture and furnishings, for each room; (b) equipment, such as pots, pans, crockery, washing machine, cooker, etc; and (c) workmanship, with regard to internal decorations, carpets, curtains, and fittings (such as cupboards). Standards must be set, such that carpets with flaws are unacceptable, as are old hospital curtains. The specified standard must be achieved before clients move into flats/homes. A set budget must be identified in situations where the purchase of household goods is required. This is likely to be greatest when a house is first being set up. The decision has to be made as to what the clients and organization should pay for, and where suitable funds are located. In practice it may be easier to get clients to contribute towards bedroom furniture through social security benefits or savings, as it can go with them when they move, particularly if a special bed or comfortable chair is used. It is easier for the housing organization to pay for and maintain communal goods, although this requires an easily implemented purchasing and replacements policy to be set up well in advance of the move.

It is unwise to rely on any social security allowances to set up the whole house, given the frequent changes in legislation and the low amounts involved. For example, in 1984–85, single payments of £400 were available in the UK for every person receiving social security wishing to set up a home for themselves. In practice, this amount barely covered bedroom furniture and bedding if good quality goods were to be purchased.

It is important to look at any purchases with an eye to quality, particularly in a staffed housing situation, where household goods are subject to that much more wear and tear, merely by the number of people using it.

Running the house

As well as having a set standard for the living environment, there must also be mechanisms by which the standard of care can be monitored.

The purpose of the home and tasks to be tackled can be defined by a house operational policy. This can be a very good way to orientate both staff and clients when they are new or lacking direction. Operational policies can vary a good deal, from being a philosophical, theoretical statement to a very practical one.

The operational policy should include: (a) a brief description of the house, number of bedrooms and state who the owner is; (b) the basis for tenant selection (e.g. people with a mental handicap who are familiar with the neighbourhood), and who can nominate them; (c) who will manage the staffing, review quality of care given to tenants, and be responsible for repairs and maintenance; (d) reference to staffing levels, if a staffed house; (e) how disputes will be handled; (f) a list of services which tenants can expect to receive from the staff, landlord and any other agencies involved in supporting the house; and (g) making changes to the operational policy. Cummings *et al.* (1989) also outline main content headings of an operational policy for a staffed house.

Prior to moving into the house, procedures and policies also need to be developed for:

1. The replacement of furniture, i.e. which is to be paid for by clients, by the housing organization or another source;
2. Housing repairs and maintenance, such as plumbing, clearing the roof gutters, repairing electrical faults;
3. The payment of bills, i.e. gas, electricity, water rates; the staff also contribute to these bills in the house, by virtue of working there, sleeping over, etc.

It is unfair to expect clients to pay for the staff's contribution to electricity, gas, etc. A system must be established by which the organization managing the staff, contributes towards the bills; 20% (or one-fifth) would seem to be a reasonable amount in a house where there are four clients.

Even the most able clients will probably need help in learning how to pay a bill, particularly if they have lived in an institution for many years. In many instances it is unrealistic to expect that the clients will ever be able to handle bill-paying independently, with care staff having to take the responsibility for handling their money. This requires procedures to be set for staff to follow and for them to be good book-keepers and absolutely scrupulous in the handling of clients' monies. It also indicates the need for this aspect of client care to be monitored regularly by an outsider, perhaps from the housing management committee (see later).

Failure to establish clear policies with regard to the above can result in low morale of clients and staff, frustrations, lack of furniture and even outstanding bills.

Monitoring standards

The purpose of monitoring the standard of accommodation and/or care clients receive is to ensure that they are receiving services suited to their needs. This requires assessment and evaluation of the facility concerned. Various 'tools' by which residential services can be evaluated are summarized by Berry (1985) and include:

1. Program Analysis of Service Systems (PASS) (Wolfensberger and Glenn, 1975) which rates facilities in terms of proximity to community services, access, size, appearance of the building, programmes run for clients, and opportunities for social integration; evaluations using PASS are carried out by four assessors;
2. Standards for Community Agencies serving Persons with Mental Retardation and other Developmental Disabilities, developed by the Joint Commission on Accreditation of Hospitals (1973) in the USA, where a detailed survey questionnaire is the basis of assessment; services which have been known to have achieved a minimum standard receive accreditation;
3. The Delphi technique (Elkins et al., 1980), which systematically processes individual judgements about problems and issues, and can be used to predict future patterns of services;
4. The checklist of standards, developed by National Development Group (1980) in the United Kingdom, which aims at: (a) identifying strengths, weaknesses and gaps in existing services, as well as improving them; (b) providing a baseline to measure progress, and a means for developing new services, and (c) educating the staff;
5. Schonell Evaluation and Accreditation Procedure (SEAP) (Andrews, Elkins and Berry, 1983) which involves the use of questionnaires and site visit to the facility.

With regard to residential service evaluations, Berry (1985) suggests that the team could comprise residential staff, parents, clients, paramedical professionals, or other experts, such as an architect. In practice it may prove useful to include people outside the service, who are as yet unbiased and may be more able to retain some objectivity. Berry notes the importance of allowing evaluators to have open access to records, staff, clients, families, etc., in order to obtain information from a range of sources.

Advisory groups and project committees

Another means by which standards in residential services may be monitored in an on-going way is through the establishment of housing advisory groups. In practice, each home/hostel could have its own advisory group, which would be available to clients and staff to help in the resolution of any difficulties, to act as a resource and would monitor standards of care received by clients, in terms of the physical environment and care received by staff.

Gathercole (1981a) suggests that such groups would be useful to clients living in unstaffed housing, and may only be needed for six months post move, with a list maintained to the housing and community worker. This may be possible in the situation where very able clients are concerned. In the case of less able clients, a housing advisory group would need to be maintained and on-going, particularly in a staffed housing situation. It would need to be more than 'advisory' and at times directive, in order to ensure clients are living in suitable accommodation and receiving the care needed.

Such groups, known as project committees, have been used extensively in the London borough of Southwark. Co-ordinated by the Southwark Mental Handicap Consortium (SMHC) (1986), the housing being developed for groups of 2–5 people, has required contributions from housing associations to build/refurbish and maintain the accommodation, and the two local health authorities to staff the houses.

Each home, or in some instances group of flats, has its own project committee. The size of committees vary, but include a representative from the housing association, the health authority, the SMHC, and other useful/local people, such as councillors, or someone from the local authority. A representative from the staff group, usually the house leader, is in attendance at meetings, and clients are welcome at any time. Occupational therapists attend when issues pertaining to design and adaptations are discussed. Other experts can be called in as required.

The tasks of the project committee vary, depending on the stage of development of the house. Prior to opening the house, committees must identify potential tenants, deal with any housing design needed or adaptations, establish an operational policy for the house, and number of staff required. The committee must ensure that the house is equipped to a basic standard before clients move in, and that all adaptations and work is complete.

After clients have moved, the committee must become involved in the resolution of any problems, such as difficulty in obtaining benefits, the need for further adaptations, or filling vacancies, should one become available. The committee is there to ensure that the guidelines as set out in the operational policy are fulfilled.

Committee meetings may vary in their frequency, from once every 6 weeks to once every 12 weeks, depending on the tasks the committee is grappling with. Meetings give an opportunity for all the organizations involved to air their views, and most importantly, for the clients and staff. Occupational therapists can contribute both as advisors on house layout and as permanent members. The broad-training and overview of clients' needs by OTs has been of particular assistance in the development of housing as well as running of houses.

SUMMARY

Various issues related to the development of housing options for people with mental handicaps have been discussed, and case examples used to illustrate different points. Undoubtedly, the OT has an enormous contribution to make in this area, particularly in the assessment and modification of houses. However, it is important that whatever input is given should be done in the context of a system that continues to review the quality and standards of accommodation clients receive.

FURTHER READING

Housing and Mental Handicap

Benson-Wilson, A. and Kendall, A. (1978) Two ordinary terraced houses in Skelmersdale adapted to house six mentally handicapped children. *Design for Special Needs,* **12**, 10-11.

Centre on Environment for the Handicapped (1985) *House Adaptations for People with a Mental Handicap*, Seminar Report, Centre on Environment for the Handicapped, London.

Department of the Environment (1983) *Housing for Mentally Ill and Mentally Handicapped People*, HMSO, London.

Dybwad, G., Ganges, A. and Gray, G.V. (1981) *Architectural Barriers and People with Mental Retardation*, National Centre for a Barrier Free Environment, Washington DC.

Heginbotham, C. (1980) Housing choice for mentally handicapped people. *Design for Special Needs*, **23**, 11-15.

McCarthy, R. (1984) Lewisham and North Southwark: putting care into the community. *Design for Special Needs*, **36**, 9-11.

Richie, J., Keegan, J. and Bosquanet, N. (1983) *Housing for Mentally Ill and Mentally Handicapped People: a Research Study of Housing Provision in England and Wales*, Department of the Environment, HMSO, London.

Shearer, A. (1978) Purpose-built units for 24 mentally handicapped children in Eastbourne, *Design for Special Needs*, **12**, 11-13.

Symons, J. (1978a) Health service provisions for mentally handicapped people. *Design for Special Needs*, **15**, 22-6.

Symons, J. (1978b) Architecture and community care – the needs of handicapped people. *Design for Special Needs*, **17**, 23-6.

Housing – General

Cantle, F.E. and Sharp, N.A. (1977) *Mobility housing for flexibility in housing for the disabled*, Centre on Environment for the Handicapped, London.

Conacher, G. (1986) *Kitchen Sense for Disabled People*, Croom Helm, London.

Department of the Environment (1977) *Wheelchair Housing: a Survey of Purpose Designed Dwellings for Disabled People*, HMSO, London.

Edgington, A. (1984) Survey of major adaptations. *British Journal of Occupational Therapy*, **47** (2), 46-9.

Foott, S. (ed.) (1976) *Kitchen Sense for Disabled and Elderly People of all Ages*, Heinemann Medical, London.

Goldsmith, S. (1974) *Mobility Housing*, Housing Development Directorate, London.

Goldsmith, S. (1976) *Designing for the Disabled*, RIBA, London.

Hale, G. (1983) *The New Source Book for the Disabled*, Heinemann, London.

Lifchez, R. and Winslow, B. (1979) *Design for Independent Living: the Environment and Physically Disabled People*, Architectural Press, London.

Lockhart, T. (1981) *Housing Adaptations for Disabled People*, Architectural Press, London.

Macdonald, S. (1978) Designing adaptations for the disabled, part 2. *British Journal of Occupational Therapy* **41** (2), 65-6.

Nichols, P., Haworth, R. and Hopkins, J. (1981) *Disabled: an Illustrated Manual of Help and Self Help*, David and Charles, London.

Page, M. and Feeney, R.J. (1980) Measurement and assessment techniques for WC and bathaids for the disabled. *Nursing Times*, August 7, 1404–8.

Penton, J. (1980) *A Handbook of Housing for Disabled People*, London Housing Consortium West Group, London.

Raschko, B.B. (1982) *Housing Interiors for the Disabled and Elderly*, Van Nostrand Rienhold, New York.

Thorpe, S. (1985a) *Access for Disabled: Design Guidelines for Developers*, Centre on Environment for the Handicapped, London.

Thorpe, S. (1985b) *Housing Design Sheets*, Centre on Environment for the Handicapped, London.

Thorpe, S. (1986) *Designing for People with Sensory Impairments*, Centre on Environment for the Handicapped, London.

6

Preparation and work with people with profound mental handicap, behaviour problems and mental illness

PROFOUND MENTAL HANDICAP

Profound mental handicap is associated with low scores on intelligence tests (e.g. IQ score below 19), little, if any, intelligible speech, often in association with sensory, skeletal and physical abnormalities – some 40% of people with profound mental handicaps are either bedridden or semi-ambulatory (Cleland, 1979). There is also a shorter than average life expectancy, largely due to associated physical complications, and a higher rate of institutionalization at an early age than less handicapped people. Various physical problems noted in the literature include spasticity and epilepsy, gynaecological and dental problems, and fecal and urinary incontinence (Cleland, 1979; Heaton-Ward and Willey, 1984).

The combination of physical problems with a limited means to communicate with others renders a state of dependence and helplessness of profoundly handicapped people. It has been suggested that frustration due to limited means of communication is linked to aggressive behaviours often observed with these clients (Cleland). Aggression towards others or oneself, both very common in this group, may also be linked to: (a) boredom, through limited options for creating 'boredom antidotes'; (b) a response to high levels of noise, and (c) a higher pain threshold, due to the impairment of one or more senses (i.e. sight, smell, touch, taste, hearing); this would mean that the individual is less able to perceive and avoid pain-inducing situations, such as hitting another person or putting a hand on an electric hotplate.

Other behaviours associated with profound handicap include: (a) pica, the eating of objects such as dirt, paint or cigarette butts, that have no nutritional value; (b) coprophagy, the ingestion of faeces;

(c) smearing of faeces in the nearby environment or on oneself; (d) rumination and vomiting of food; (e) extreme anxiety; and (f) stereotyped movements, such as body rocking, which are self-stimulating (Cleland).

Both Brudenell (1986) and Cleland emphasize the range of emotions and social interactions that profoundly handicapped people are able to show, including smiling, humour, touching, and social interest in others.

Hospital or community housing

There are many and varying views with regard to community versus hospital care for people with profound mental handicap and for severe behaviour problems.

Pro-community views

In addition to normalization philosophy and increasing contact with the community, the trend towards community placement has been based, in part, on the assumption that small community residences will provide environments more conducive to increasing 'adaptive competence' than those found in institutional settings (Silverman et al., 1986). It has been suggested that the movement to community facilities from hospitals will result in positive developmental outcome for all people, regardless of the degree of handicap (Menolascino and McGee, 1981). The little research that has been done on the impact of de-institutionalization on people with profound handicaps does support his suggestion, although only small samples were used or the subjects' functional levels were not detailed sufficiently (O'Neill et al., 1985).

However, both O'Neill et al. (1985), Rawlings (1985a,b), and Thomas et al. (1986), were able to substantiate through their studies that people with profound handicaps living in community houses spend more time engaged in 'appropriate' activities (such as activities of daily living, leisure pursuits and educational programmes) than people with the same disabilities living in institutions. The latter spent more time engaged in inappropriate activities such as self-stimulation, aggressive behaviour or attention-seeking behaviour. In the community there was a reduction in stereotyped behaviours (such as rocking) amongst subjects, as well as increased staff–client interaction, which were resident oriented. Rawlings

(1985b) suggests that this fact, and the independence given to staff by their management, allowed subjects to do things when they wanted, which led to a reduction in boredom and frustration. O'Neill *et al.* (1985) noted that people with profound handicaps living outside the hospital spent more time engaged in an array of community activities, than they ever had. Saxby *et al.* (1986) showed that whilst using shops, cafes and public houses, this client group were able to engage in activities appropriate to the setting, and most had contact with some members of the community. The shop owners and shop staff concerned were happy for the clients to use their facilities; inappropriate behaviours occurred approximately 10% of the time in shops and 15% in cafes or pubs.

The studies did not result in confirming the hypothesis that the skills of clients would be enhanced in the community as against hospital setting despite: (a) an increase in appropriate behaviour, and (b) more interaction between staff and clients. Researchers have suggested that the learning potential of severely and profoundly handicapped people may be very limited indeed. (Ellis *et al.*, 1982).

What the studies infer overall is that people with profound and severe mental handicaps can benefit in terms of day-to-day activity patterns and have an improved quality of life, when living in supportive community housing and that this is a realistic goal. Further to this, Cummings *et al.* (1989) demonstrates that it is possible to maintain people with challenging behaviours in ordinary, community housing.

Pro-hospital views

By contrast, other researchers view the movement of people with profound handicaps into the community (from institutions) as an unrealistic goal, which would not improve quality of life, put individuals at risk and not enhance the development of skills (Ellis *et al.*, 1981). Furthermore, Eyman (1976), Close (1977) and Silverman *et al.* (1986) observed that living in the community was of no advantage in terms of skill acquisition for this client group. This result has been used as an argument against the establishment of community houses for people with profound handicaps. But, as Rawlings (1985b) suggests, skill acquisition as an index of quality of care should be reconsidered, given the suggestion that the learning potential among severely and profoundly handicapped people may be very limited (Ellis *et al.*, 1982).

Strong views have been stated in support of the on-going use of residual mental handicap hospital units or specialist units for those clients who are severely/profoundly handicapped or have behaviour problems (DHSS, 1971; Shapiro, 1974; Day, 1983; Reid, 1983; Heaton-Ward and Willey, 1984). It has also been suggested that the hospitals could be used: (a) as a venue for training potential community staff; (b) as centres for diagnostic and assessment services, and (c) for staff reinforcement and support and professional consultation (Martin, 1974).

Livingstone (1987) suggested that hospitals (a) have existing facilities such as community halls, workshops and treatment centres and have potential for redevelopment; (b) are the logical focal point for the co-ordination of all forms of residential care, and (c) can and should be a source of help for community clients in terms of investigative help, day facilities, and as a haven in times of need.

By comparison, Keene and James (1986) speak out strongly against the establishment of specialist units for people with profound mental handicaps or behavioural problems, maintaining that such settings create problems, for both staff and client alike. The unit they describe had high staffing ratios, and because it was associated with a hospital, had the benefit of centralized laundry, cooking and domestic services, which enabled the nurses to have more time with clients. However, several problems emerged: (a) beds became blocked as community facilities were unwilling to take on the burden of a 'difficult' client; (b) there were fewer opportunities to be involved in the development of living skills because these tasks were being dealt with by the hospital services, and (c) the existence of the unit tended to create an intolerance of moderately disruptive behaviour and a reluctance to attempt to solve individuals' problems other than by removing them to the 'Behavioural Unit'.

A similar unit for people with profound handicaps within the same complex proved bad for staff morale, which led to a high staff turnover because they were barely able to cope with dealing with the basic demands of toileting, feeding, etc. of clients and were unable to develop other occupational or therapeutic programmes. The authors maintain that the individuals in the units mentioned could be supported in ordinary community housing. However, they fail to detail how this could be achieved!

A range of options

It is difficult to make sense of the conflicting views mentioned. Of course, community housing is preferable for people with profound mental handicap and/or severe behavioural problems, but the features of such programmes need to be carefully structured.

Thomas *et al.* (1986) attribute the success of their community programme for people with profound handicaps to: (a) improved staff-client ratios; (b) greater physical integration of the setting into the community; (c) smaller facility size; (d) differences in architectural design; (e) improved client access to different activity areas; (f) grater material enrichment; (g) improved autonomy over budget use and staff recruitment; and (h) increased permanence of staff allocation in the community settings. Saxby *et al.* (1986) point to the importance of: (a) physical appearance of clients, in terms of quality and adult appropriateness of clothing and hairstyle; (b) competence of staff; (c) uses of amenities in small groups; and (d) the fact that the clients were genuine customers and 'contributing to the economy', in the integration and acceptance of people with profound handicaps in public places, such as shops, public bars and cafes. These and other factors, important to the success of community programmes for this client group will be expanded upon in the next two sections of the chapter.

Despite the vehement arguments of Keene and James, specialized units perhaps have a role, although this needs to be carefully defined. The use of former institutions for this purpose is not very desirable, and perhaps such services could be set up in ordinary housing, with the necessary specialist staff in place. Studies by McBrien (1987) and Fidura, Lindsey and Walker (1987) illustrate the use of behavioural units for day attendance or as a short-term in-patient facility in maintaining people with severe behaviour problems in the community in the long term. Also described in the literature is the use of a specialised multidisciplinary community team used to support people with severe mental handicap and problem behaviours in the community (Emerson, *et al.*, 1988; Toogood, *et al.*, 1988).

Living in the community–OT involvement

The importance of involvement in constructive activity in reducing self-injurous and stereotypic behaviours has been noted by many researchers (Favell, 1973; Mulick *et al.*, 1978; Horner, 1980; Lockwood and Bourland, 1982). This would indicate great opportunities for OT input and participation with such clients.

The aim of this section is to list the wide variety of approaches and activities that OTs can use when working with people with profound mental handicap and/or behaviour problems. Readers should consult the papers cited for details as to how to set up and implement programmes.

The previous discussion in Chapter 2 relating to preparation prior to leaving hospital applies to profoundly handicapped people also. For illustrations, see Felce and Toogood (1988), Toogood *et al*. (1988), and the case study of David (Case Study B) in Appendix 1. For information on assessment as applied to this client group, see Chapters 3, 4 and 5.

Structured daily routine Low levels of purposeful activity amongst clients with severe and profound mental handicap living in a variety of facilities or attending day programmes have been observed by various researchers Porterfield, Blunden and Blewitt, 1980; Mansell *et al*., 1982). They considered that if such clients were to develop any skills or be receptive to their environment then the staff would have to organize activities in such a way so as to promote client engagement.

Room management techniques were found to lead clients spending more time engaged in purposeful activity or in interactions with other people (McBrien and Weightman, 1980; Porterfield, Blunden and Blewitt, 1980; Mansell *et al*., 1982). (Room management involves one staff member taking on the role of prompting clients to get involved in constructive activities, with another dealing specifically with the needs of individuals (e.g. to go to the toilet) and deal with any visitors. Other staff, if available, do individual or group work with clients. Clients were presented with a range of leisure type activities, such as crafts, puzzles, and simple art.) McCool *et al*. (1989) describe and illustrate the use of goal setting for clients to provide them, and care staff a daily structure, and as a means of replacing destructive behaviour with constructive activity.

A similar attempt to structure the activities of clients and staff could be to use a 24-hour detailed routine in staffed housing. All daily activities can be included in such routines – personal care, cooking, domestic duties – indeed, Mansell *et al*. (1984) have noted that involvement in domestic activities are very effective in the promotion of 'engaged behaviour' of people with profound mental handicaps living in staffed housing.

The structure for each hour of the day could be looked at in 'blocks', with an activity assigned, appropriate to the individual concerned. The length of the time block will depend on the disability of the client, and for more disabled people timing might need to be broken down into 15-minute blocks. For example:

8.00– 8.15 a.m. – get out of bed; go to toilet, have bath/shower
8.15– 8.30 a.m. – bath/shower continued; get dressed
8.30– 8.45 a.m. – prepare, eat breakfast

8.45 – 9.00 a.m. – eat breakfast continued; wash up breakfast dishes
9.00 – 9.15 a.m. – finish breakfast dishes, make bed, tidy room
9.15 – 9.30 a.m. – go shopping
9.30 – 9.45 a.m. – shopping
9.45 –10.00 a.m. – shopping
10.00 –10.15 a.m. – unpack shopping, make drink if needed
10.15 –10.30 a.m. – OT visit – activities, etc.

It is important not to be too rigid about the activities and their timing. Such routines ensure that time of the individual and staff is defined. It is particularly useful when staff feel that an individual's needs and demands are overwhelming, and they do not know where to start.

There is great scope for OTs to be involved in the planning, structure and incorporation of stimulating activities in such programmes. It requires assessment of an individual's skills and interests (Chapter 3) and access to necessary equipment.

Importance of constructive activity Research findings indicating the importance of involvement in constructive activity in the reduction of self-injurious and stereotypic behaviours (Warren and Burns, 1970; Favell, 1973; Mulick *et al.*, 1978; Horner, 1980; Lockwood and Bourland, 1982), would suggest that there is great need for OT input with such clients.

Self-injurious behaviour Approaches to dealing with self-injurious behaviour include the use of drugs, physical restraints, punishment, over-correction, time-out, reinforcers, and consistent approaches to the individual by care staff, parents, friends, etc. (Stephens and Allen, 1967; Foxx and Dufrense, 1984; Murphy and Wilson, 1985; Halpern and Andrasik, 1986; Matson and Gorman-smith, 1986). However, it has been noted that these various techniques, particularly time-out, can only be used successfully in the context of an enriched environment, activities and reinforcement of alternative (non-injurious) behaviour (Thomas and Howard, 1971; Lockwood and Bourland, 1982; Foxx and Dufrense, 1984; Mander and Lyon, 1988). This is well illustrated in case study form by these authors, where the availability and involvement in activities contributed significantly in the reduction of head banging, fingerpicking, self-biting and hitting. Lockwood and Bourland particularly note the importance of structuring the environment to engender and maintain toy use. In their study, this meant that the toys had to be attached by an elasticized line to a metal hanger, fixed to the wheelchair the subjects were sitting in; in the situation when toys were not fixed and the subjects threw the toys out of reach, they began to self-injure again.

The significance of the relationship developed between client and therapist in the development of skills and reduction of self-injury has also been noted (Thomas and Howard). The building of a relationship between client and therapist enabled the client to develop an interest in his environment and develop skills needed to control it.

Hyperactivity Similar to the management of self-injurious behaviour, approaches to dealing with hyperactivity in people with mental handicap include the use of drugs, punishment, time-out, physical restraints and reinforcement procedures (Whitman, Caponigri and Mercurio, 1971). In their study, these authors modify the subject's behaviour with reinforcement procedures in conjunction with audio, visual and tactile stimulation.

Smearing of faeces Traditional approaches to the management of smearing includes isolation or seclusion, physical restraint and operant conditioning (Cleland, 1979). Despite the repulsiveness of such behaviour, Cleland suggests that smearing is a form of communication, and may be channelled into a more socially acceptable form. He suggests that if an individual who smears is to be placed in a seclusion room, elimination of the more obnoxious aspects of this habit may be managed by: (a) leaving a pile of non-toxic paint, similar in colour and consistency to faecal matter, in the room for the person to 'paint' with; and (b) making sure that the walls are painted with a surface that is easily washable. The overall objective would be that the individual would be able to transfer to an acceptable substitute for faeces, and perhaps even incorporate several colours!

Unfortunately there have been no formal studies to test this plan. However, Cleland notes the study of Stockton (1973), who compared the receptiveness of smearers and non-smearers to finger paint that was the consistency of faeces, and found that all the smearers readily painted with this medium, as against half of the non-smearers, and 'acted like artists'.

OT and activities

The result of these studies are of particular relevance to OTs involved in using activities with people exhibiting very disturbed behaviour(s).

1. Age appropriateness of activities In normalization terms, when it is suggested that activities must be age appropriate, it may appear to be most unsatisfactory for toys to be used in relation to adults (Mulick *et al.*, 1978; Lockwood and Bourland, 1982). However, this attitude fails to recognize where client's skills are on a developmental continuum, and perhaps activities which he finds stimulating, which do not seem appropriate to his age. Respect for clients can be shown in the way in which the therapist speaks to and interacts with the client, enabling any activity to be presented in an age-appropriate manner. Given this, the use of toys and sensory activities is indicated, provided that clients can be seen to: (a) benefit, in terms of developing manipulative/cognitive/other skills; (b) enjoy the activity, and (c) are given direction by the therapist to develop beyond the activity.

2. Activity as a substitute for undesirable behaviour Activities can be skilfully selected by the therapist to provide a satisfying substitute for an undesirable behaviour. For example, Lockwood and Bourland (1982) selected colourful rubber and soft plastic toys that could be chewed, because they were thought to provide intraoral and proprioceptive stimuli similar to those arising from finger biting. Finger biting was a behaviour they were attempting to eliminate. Similarly, Stockton (1973) uses fingerpaint as a substitute for faeces. In both cases, the unwanted behaviour has been channelled into some kind of constructive activity.

3. Activities that are meaningful to the individual It is important for the OT to be able to match activities according to the interests of the individual, in order to provide something meaningful to him or her.

For example, Thomas and Howard (1971) observed that a client who was a head banger enjoyed playing in the bath. They were able to divert his attention away from this by using a whirlpool bath as part of his activity sessions.

Having been able to engage the client, the therapist must then be able to go on to help the client develop other skills in order to manipulate and control his environment. In the example above, as the client's head banging reduced and restraints were removed, the therapist was able to help him develop self-help skills before and after the bath.

4. Building on the individual's skills The therapist must also aim to capitalize on any skills the client does have, and direct this into constructive activity. For example, Stockton (1973) was able to direct the skill of spinning a coin into spinning a top, flicking the wheel of a spinning wheel, and spinning a ball suspended from the ceiling or a rail above the person's head. Ripping one's own clothes might be transferred to ripping up newspapers or cardboard, in the process of recycling paper.

Following the principle of individual skill and interest, various activities may be devised, or toys developed. This has been done by Phoebe Caldwell (1985) who has developed a range of toys based on the interests of some of the profoundly handicapped people with whom she has worked.

Activities that OTs working with people with profound handicaps often use include gross and fine motor activities, sensory experiences and leisure. For discussion on training in living skills with special reference to profound handicap, see Chapter 4. For further reading, see Hogg and Sebba (1986a,b) and Critchley (1989).

ADL There are many and varied programmes already established for the teaching of ADL skills to people with severe and profound mental handicap. These are listed at the end of the chapter, and there is further detailed discussion on ADL in Chapter 6.

Gross and fine motor skills Programmes to develop the motor skills of adults and children with a range of physical disabilities are many and varied. Those of particular use to people with an additional mental handicap are noted in Table 6.1. See also Chu (1989) for comparison of Bobath, Ayres, and conductive education approaches to cerebral palsy. Techniques not noted include the Fay–Doman–Delacato Neuromuscular Reflex Therapy, Proprioceptive Neuromuscular Facilitation (PNF) and the Brunstrom Approach, because of the difficulty in application to people with mental handicaps due to: (a) the number of staff/carers required to provide constant input, which can be difficult to achieve in the institutional setting, let alone in the community when resources are dispersed (Fay–Doman–Delacato method), and (b) emphasis on verbal commands which would be difficult for a person with poor comprehension to understand (PNF and Brunstrom Approach) (Lederman, 1984).

In some situations, the development of motor skills may be seen as the domain of the physiotherapist. None the less, OTs need to be able to use principles such as Reflex Inhibiting Positions (RIPs) or sensory stimulation in order to enable independence of individuals in daily living tasks or participation in other activities in daily living tasks or participation in other activities of interest (Chia, 1985).

Table 6.1 Gross and fine motor skills programmes

Author	Techniques
Presland (1982)	Physical guidance; positioning; special seating; following developmental sequence; using reinforcers
Finnie (1974)	Control of reflexes through handling and positioning; use of equipment and positioning for various aspects of ADL, fine motor function and play
Bobath (1978)	Suppression of abnormal patterns of movement and introduction of normal patterns by using reflex inhibiting movement patterns and 'key points of control'
Rood (1962)	Sensory stimulation - light touching, brushing, stroking, vibration, joint compression, stretch, resistance, developmental sequencing of functional activities, movement patterns and individual muscle groups
Ayres (1972)	Integration of sensory stimuli and reflexes to produce neural organization through series of graded activities; use of standardized tests and subjective clinical impressions

The decision to use one approach or another will invariably depend on the presenting problems of the individual concerned, as well as the ease with which it can be applied in the community setting. For this reason, techniques which are 'portable', requiring minimal or no equipment (for example Rood or Bobath) are very easily applied in the home setting. Furthermore, the availability of training will also affect which techniques can be used. This is particularly the case with setting up sensory integration programmes.

Regardless of the techniques used, therapists must ensure that carers are taught how to apply them. This is an obvious point to make, but can be quite difficult to achieve in a staffed housing situation where staff work in shifts. This emphasizes the importance of teaching handling techniques in introduction or in-service training programmes for care staff, reinforced by written guidelines and follow-up in the home.

It is very important for OTs working in the community and encountering people with mental handicaps with additional physical disability, to receive training in handling and treatment techniques. In practice, however, OTs tend to use an eclectic approach; this is well illustrated by Ledermen (1984), whose approach to motor development is summarized in Table 6.2.

It may be that achievements in motor development for an

Table 6.2 Summary of activities/approaches to develop motor skills as suggested by Lederman (1984)

Motor problem	Activities
Hypotonus	Facilitation techniques - use of fast irregular rhythms to stimulate muscle tone, e.g. icing, vestibular stimulation, vibration, quick stretch, tapping, joint compression, resistance
Hypertonus	Inhibition techniques to decrease muscle tone, e.g. neutral warmth, slow vestibular stimulation, slow rocking and rolling, slow stroking, pressure on insertion of muscle, light joint compression, maintainted speech, cold. Use of equipment such as a waterbed and electromyographic feedback
Muscle strength	Graded exercise - passive, active assistive, active, resistance
Endurance	Grading of activities to involve moderate resistance, greater number of repetitions, greater length of time
Range of motion	Relaxation, active stretching, passive stretching
Gross motor skills, head control	Prone position on a wedge; scooter board activities in prone position; posture vest with weighted shoulders; sensory feedback techniques
Rolling	Passive rotation of trunk; waterbeds; sensory air flow mats; rolling in a barrel
Creeping and crawling	Encourage head extension and weight bearing on forearms through placing person on wedge in prone position; weight bearing on extended arms and legs, on floor or vestibular board, whilst being gently rocked by therapist; scooter board activities; crawling tunnels, barrel crawls, crawling obstacle courses
Sitting	Activities to improve trunk rotation; assistance to sitting from supine, e.g. individual holds onto towel or broom handle whilst therapist pulls; practice sitting on various objects; prescription of special chairs
Standing	Use of prone standers or standing tables during activities
Advanced skills	Jumping on a trampoline, from one place to another; walking up stairs; using bicycles, tricycles; climbing on surfaces of different heights, ball games; walking on stilts
Fine motor skills	Activities to provide awareness of hands, e.g. using nail polish, tactile stimulation. Activities to encourage reach, e.g. reaching toys, interesting objects; practicing various grasps, along developmental sequence, i.e. palmar grasp to pincer and opposition. Activities include doing puzzles, stringing beads, finger puppets, unscrewing nuts and bolts, pen and paper tasks

individual may be limited, in which case the therapist needs to select appropriate aids to daily living. There is clearly a wide range of equipment to select from but with more physically disabled individuals the therapist should consider using switches to enable environmental control. A range of switches and how they may be assembled are described by Oke (1986).

A reading list at the end of the chapter lists useful references in the mobility training and development area.

Activities A wide range of activities can be used in order to stimulate interest in the environment and develop cognitive and sensory skills with profoundly handicapped people.

Sensory integrative activities have been found to contribute to sensory gains made by profoundly handicapped adults (Behan, 1979; Close, Carpenter and Cibri, 1986). The findings of Harrison *et al.* (1966) indicate that a combination of music and exercise can have a significant, positive effect upon the psychomotor ability of people with profound and severe handicaps.

A wide range of activities encompassing the use of water, sand, art, music and equipment to develop the sensory skills and awareness of people with profound mental handicap have been described by other authors (Norris, 1982; Ledermen, 1984; Brudenell 1986).

Programmes involving the use of computers for people with mental handicaps have been implemented successfully (Saunders, 1980; Johnson and Garrie, 1985; Armstrong and Rennie, 1986; Cromwell, 1986; Todman 1987). Given further simplification and suitable hand controls (Armstrong and Rennie), no doubt programmes could also be modified for the most profoundly handicapped individual.

Leisure Leisure can be seen to be an advanced form of social play, and requires the individual to be able to implement a combination of social, motor and cognitive skills, as well as an ability to manipulate and interact with objects and people in his environment (Ledermen, 1984). Furthermore, leisure skills have their basis in those experiences and skills acquired through childhood play.

It has been noted that individuals with profound mental handicap usually display low levels of 'free play', and because of this, may never progress to 'advanced social play' (Wehman and Marchant, 1978).

However, these researchers found that a training programme using instructions, modelling, physical guidance and verbal reinforcement

Table 6.3 Interest in activities as indicated by toy play and activities around the house

Likes	Possible activity
Baths	Swimming; using a jacuzzi
Listening to music	Making music, movement to music
Rocking/swaying	Movement to music, trampolining
Touching different textures	Cooking, gardening (both very structured); art activities – leaf, roller, potato and hand print; finger painting; collage
Throwing things	Skittles, ball games

resulted in a marked increase in independent and social play with severely handicapped children. Toys which 'act back' when played with were found to facilitate free play. Busy boxes, stacking blocks, jack-in-the-boxes, spinning tops, music boxes, rattles, balls with gravel inside and plastic squeeze boxes were identified by Wehman and Marchant to be toys particularly liked by their subjects. Keogh *et al.* (1984) were able to teach board games using vocal and physical prompts to pairs of severely handicapped adolescents.

Identifying leisure activities for people who are profoundly handicapped relies on carers/therapists to observe the individual's reaction to the activity, given the absence of a verbal response.

With regard to profoundly handicapped individuals, Ledermen suggests that the OT should concentrate on developing play skills, by trying out various activities and toys and identifying those which the individual likes. Given this, it may then be possible to use these activities to help the individual develop constructive play skills, which would include problem solving, conceptualization, fine motor skills and toy use. While this may be relevant in the setting of an OT department in a hospital or centre, in the home setting, the OT will have to identify leisure/play activities that are available in the community, if the profoundly handicapped individual is not to be isolated in the home. The Daytime Activities Questionnaire (see Appendix 2) lists various activities that could be worked through systematically in order to identify those enjoyed by the individual.

Alternatively, the individual's response to various toys or play equipment or the degree of participation in various household activities may also indicate activities that could be pursued. Some suggestions are listed in Table 6.3.

MENTAL ILLNESS AND MENTAL HANDICAP

Incidence and range of illnesses

People with mental handicaps are as vulnerable to the same range of emotional, behavioural and psychiatric disorders as the rest of the population. The presence of mental handicap may, in fact, make such people even more susceptible to emotional and psychiatric disturbances, because of structural brain abnormalities or brain damage, determined by genetic, infective, toxic or traumatic causes and the effect of handicap on lifestyle and interpersonal relationships are seen to contribute to this vulnerability (Reid, 1985). Other factors such as being 'labelled' mentally handicapped, limited bonding opportunities with parents (due to hospitalization or rejection), being sent away from the family temporarily or permanently, denial of sexuality, communication difficulties, low frustration threshold, additional physical handicaps, few opportunities for self-determination, unattractive appearance and poor personal habits have also been identified (Bouras, 1986).

The Camberwell study clearly illustrates the range of mental illnesses apparent in adults with mental handicap (Corbett, 1979). Psychiatric diagnosis was made on 46% of subjects (Table 6.4), although the past history of schizophrenia and manic depressive psychosis was likely to be an underestimate. (Corbett attributes this to the inadequacy of hospital records and the strict criteria used in the study.)

In addition to those listed on Table 6.4, other psychiatric disorders associated with mental handicap include autism, and hyperkinetic syndromes, as well as acute and chronic organic brain syndromes, and neurotic, conduct and personality disorders (Reid). Bouras, Drummond, Brooks and Laws (1988) observed that there were wide variations in the incidence of mental illness amongst people with mental handicaps, in recent studies. This ranged from 14.3% of subjects in a study by Eaton and Menolascino (1982) in Nebraska, 27% of subjects in a study by Lund (1985) in Denmark and 85% of a sample of 130 people referred to an outpatient mental health clinic in Chicago (Benson, 1985)! Bouras et al. (1988) note the methodological differences between the studies. In their own study, they found an incidence of mental illness in 42.06% of subjects (n = 233), a reasonable comparison to Corbett's. Bouras et al. (1988) also noted a lower incidence of psychiatric diagnosis with severity of handicap, presumably related to the difficulties in assessing mental illness in clients with limited communication skills.

Table 6.4 Psychiatric disorder in adults with mental handicap; the Camberwell study

Psychiatric disorder	No.	%
No disorder	216	54
Past history of schizophrenia	11	3
Current schizophrenia	14	3.5
Past history of depression/manic depressive psychosis	8	2
Current depressive illness	7	2
Current manic depressive psychosis	6	1.5
Symptoms of childhood psychosis	33	8
Behaviour disorder	102	25
Other	5	1
Total	402	100

Note: Ss in community = 137
      Ss in hospital = 265
      Total Ss = 402

In general, there is a tendency for all types of mental illness to decrease with age (Corbett), with the exception of organic disorders (Reid). However, James (1986) has observed an increased incidence in affective disorders and persistence of behavioural problems amongst older people with mental handicaps. Bouras and Drummond (1989) observed that older people with mental handicaps tend to be referred for psychiatric assessment either when cognitive function deteriorates due to age, as in middle-aged adults with Down's Syndrome, or when elderly parents are no longer able to care for them.

Difficulties in diagnosis

Many authors confirm difficulties in diagnosing mental illnesses of people with mental handicaps (Reid, 1972; Corbett, 1979; Wright, 1982; Bouras, 1986; Sireling, 1986). The use of existing diagnostic categories to describe personality disorders with these clients is inadequate, as is the difficulty in determining psychosis in severely and profoundly handicapped people, where very florid symptoms must be exhibited if a diagnosis of schizophrenia is to be made (Corbett). It is extremely difficult to diagnose a depressive illness in a person who does not speak (Sireling). Distinguishing mental illness from abnormal behaviour is also important (Bouras).

In those clients with no speech or communication system, behavioural observations of caretakers are given more weight in the diagnosis process (Bouras), although Menolascino, Gilson and Levitas (1986) caution that the clinical history may be 'shaped' by these persons.

131

Manifestation of psychiatric illnesses

Often the manifestation of psychiatric illnesses in people with mental handicaps differs from the norm, and this is well illustrated by case examples (Reid, 1972; Heaton-Ward, 1976; Corbett, 1979; Reid, 1985; Bouras, 1986; Menolascino, Gilson and Levitas, 1986). Some of these as described by the above authors are noted below:

1. Reactive depression, a common response to the loss of a significant caregiver or placement in an institution, may be manifested in regressed behaviour, such as wetting and soiling, aggression, self-mutilation or disturbances of eating and sleeping. Feelings of despair, hopelessness and guilt may be reported concretely in terms of a fear that caretakers, family, etc, no longer love the client, and suicidal ideation, in terms of increased fearfulness, and dependence to the point of clinging (Menolascino, Gilson and Levitas, 1986).

   In his study of elderly residents in a mental handicap institution, James (1986) noted that depression in elderly subjects presented as: (a) over-concern about bodily function, varying in severity from persistent complaints about constipation to nihilistic delusions, and (b) social withdrawal. Direct expressions of unhappiness were not commonly reported. Suggested triggers of affective disorders amongst these subjects included: (a) loss or threat of loss of close friends by death, or movements to another home; and (b) chronic physical illness or handicap, which caused individuals to abandon long-cherished hopes of discharge and return to their home area.

2. Anxiety may be confused with over-activity; the person may be irritable, aggressive, lose weight, sleep badly, and appear to be rigid and stubborn (Bouras).

3. Hypochondriacal symptoms may be a form of attention seeking (Bouras).

4. Functional psychoses may present in the form of loss of living skills, or withdrawal fearfulness, sleep disorder, and hallucinations, without a complex delusional system (Heaton-Ward).

5. The presentation of affective psychoses with mood swings between hypomania and psychotic depression, may take the form of eating and sleeping disturbances. A spending spree may consist of spending all of a tiny allowance (in a institution) and grandiosity by insistence that one is not retarded, and can do something well beyond one's capabilities (Menolascino, Gilson and Levitas).

OT input

It is important for OTs to appreciate the outward manifestations of psychiatric illnesses, given their unusual exhibition, particularly in the form of loss of skills. The OT may find him/herself being referred clients to deal with exhibiting some of these 'behaviours', in which case he/she needs to be able to identify the appropriate action to take. This is particularly important for the therapist working in the community, who has to deal with a variety of problems in clients, and who may be the only 'therapeutic' contact a client and his/her family has had for some time.

Example 1: A client was referred to the OT for assistance in domestic skills training; she had been coping with the preparation of breakfast and lunch and cleaning the house, but in the last few weeks had been unable to do these tasks. Her parents reported that she was eating poorly and waking up very early in the morning (4.00 a.m.), although she normally slept well (till 7.30 a.m.). the OT visited the client at home on three occasions to help practice domestic routines. Although the client was able to do the task when prompted by the OT, she was unable to perform them between visits. Subsequent discussion of this situation with a psychiatrist revealed the possibility of the client being depressed, whereupon psychiatric intervention was organized.

Example 2: The OT was involved in organizing accommodation for an elderly lady, with some independence skills, but retiring personality. (She was moving from a long stay in hospital into community housing as the hospital was closing.) The care workers helping to prepare the lady continued to emphasize the importance of the client living in a property with at least two toilets, as she spent so much time there, and was very preoccupied by her bowel movements. A suitable property that met the lady's needs in general, was identified and it indeed had two toilets. This issue was raised at a case conference, whereupon the psychiatrist pointed out that there was a possibility that the client was depressed, and worried by the move from the hospital. Intervention was then organized.

Given an understanding of the client's illness and problem, the OT in the community can pursue the client's programme as required, whether this involves training in ADL, helping the client to use community services, such as a library, or joining a club, etc. Having a psychiatric illness does not alter the content of programme that the OT implements, but gives the therapist some more information about the individual's preoccupations, so that tasks can be reorganized to be less demanding or stressful if need be.

The admission of the client to hospital does not release the community OT from her work with the client completely. It is important that detailed information about the client's skills, lifestyle and interests be passed on to the clinical staff, in order that appropriate 'in-patient' programmes are designed to build on the client's abilities and support her/his weaknesses.

Admission to hospital is also an excellent opportunity to re-assess the client's skills in a neutral environment, whether this be done by the hospital or community OT or both. Smith (1983) describes an in-patient programme in a psychiatric hospital for people with mental handicaps, based on gross motor movement experience and task-orientated groups. The programmes organized along these lines gave clients an opportunity to be involved in a variety of situations where old skills could be practised, new ones learnt, in a setting where there was little chance of failure.

Given the circumstances, the community OT should be involved in: (a) visiting the client; (b) joining the client in one or two groups; (c) being involved in the running of a group or individual sessions with the client; (d) attending any relevant case conferences; (e) the discharge planning, and (f) reviewing whether community OT input should be continued, and if so, how.

What follows is an extensive case study, included to illustrate the various ways that the community OT can constructively support clients who are mentally ill, in addition to being mentally handicapped. The importance of attending to the various behaviours and signals given off by the client is also emphasized.

Case example

Mary, a woman in her mid 50s, was referred to the CMHT for assistance in developing self-help skills and leisure interests. She lived with her 90-year-old mother in a ground floor council flat and was visited fortnightly by her sister-in-law, who also did their shopping and banking. Other services involved in supporting Mary included:

1. A GP who visited every 6–8 weeks, to see both Mary and her mother;
2. A social worker who visited weekly, and organized social security benefits and council sponsored holidays for both women, and Mary's attendance at an ATC two days a week. She had tried to

broach the issue of where Mary would live when her mother died although encountered a lot of resistance from both women whenever this was raised.

3. An Activity Therapy Centre where Mary attended two days a week, where she spent time doing various assembly jobs in the workshop, joined in outings and went to a weekly craft and adult literacy class at a nearby Adult Education Centre.

4. The home help service provided an escort service to help Mary to get to and from the collection point for the ATC bus. (Mary was fearful of crossing roads on her own, and would not venture outside the house without someone to hold on to.)

Early observations and OT aims Mary was independent in her own personal care and grooming, and routinely did the dusting, vacuuming, sweeping and tidying up in the house. She liked watching TV, knitting and reading romantic novels. However, Mary was afraid to go outside on her own, which prevented her from developing shopping, money handling and public transport skills. Because of this, Mary's sister-in-law did their shopping, which she dropped off on her fortnightly visits.

Despite her skills, Mary appeared to be a nervous person, often anxious that she might do something wrong. She was very worried about the future, and often complained of her mother's forgetfulness and deafness.

Bearing these factors in mind, as well as the goals of the social worker, the OT decided to work on: (a) structuring Mary's week; (b) developing cooking, shopping, and money-handling skills, and (c) encouraging Mary in her leisure pursuits, whilst continuing to liaise with the other agencies involved in maintaining Mary in the community.

OT activities Working with Mary was shared by the OT and community support worker from the CMHT. Mary was visited twice weekly for 1–2 hours. She was involved in the following tasks:

1. Shopping and preparing a simple meal (1 session);
2. Going for a walk (to get her out of the house, and develop confidence outdoors), talking about her knitting and reading, and what she had been up to that week (1 session). To help Mary to structure her time, a timetable was drawn up, listing various activities Mary liked to do (Table 6.5). She was asked to tick off when she had done the activity, and each week the sheet was reviewed, and praise given accordingly.

Table 6.5 Mary's timetable (* denotes reminder to do the activity on a particular day

	Monday	Tuesday	Wednes-day	Thurs-day	Friday	Satur-day	Sunday
Dust	*				*		
Vacuum	*				*		
Sweep	*				*		
Wash up							
Knit							
Read							
Make tea							

Additionally, the OT helped Mary to get to the ATC on the days she overslept or was reluctant to go. This was a very high priority, as it gave Mary opportunities to socialize, and helped reduce the tension between her and the mother.

Importance of observation   Mary had many unusual sayings, such as 'I haven't got a head/body' or 'Everything's all wrong', which often emerged if she was experiencing some difficulty in a task. However, the OT was noticing during the visits the increased frequency with which the sayings were used, which was also reported by Mary's mother. Mary was refusing to go to the ATC, her concentration had deteriorated and was eating very little. On visits coinciding with mealtimes, Mary was observed to be spitting out her food, yelling at her mother, constantly repeating her sayings and looked very unkept. The consulting psychiatrist who looked after Mary was informed, and thought it necessary to hospitalize her. She was diagnosed as having a depressive illness.

OT involvement during the in-patient phase   Mary spent 8 weeks in a small in-patient psychiatric unit in a general hospital. Her agitation settled after a few weeks in the unit which was attributed in part to medication but mostly to the stimulation offered by the unit, by way of activities and people, in contrast to her very quiet life at home. She was an active participant in cooking, craft and board games sessions. Although she was a very quiet person Mary took a keen interest in the problems of others in the unit, and would talk about this very animatedly with her own visitors.

The community OT maintained her involvement with Mary during this time in the following ways:

1. Passing on relevant information with regard to Mary's skills and interests to the staff, her fear of crossing roads, of being outside on her own, and of what the future held for her.
2. Weekly visits to Mary, which sometimes included a walk to the kiosk to buy a magazine or playing a game of dominoes.
3. Attendance at ward rounds, and involvement in planning her discharge, which required review of previous OT programmes and reassessment of Mary's needs.

It was clear Mary needed more contact with people and opportunities to go out of the house, and the question of her future accommodation had to be addressed. Visits by the OT and community support worker were to continue to develop Mary's independence skills, and leisure interests that would be particularly useful in a hostel setting. Alongside this, the social worker was to increase Mary's day centre attendance and search for suitable hostel accommodation.

Return to the community The OT and community support worker continued their twice-weekly visits, doing the following:

1. Shopping and meal preparation (1 visit);
2. Going for a walk, helping Mary to fill her pill box (and checking that she had been taking her medication), and filling in her weekly activity chart (which noted times that the OT/Support worker and her sister-in-law visited, and days she was going to the ATC);
3. Getting Mary to the ATC on the days she was not ready when the home help came; on average, Mary managed to get to the ATC two or three times a week.

Mary continued to gain confidence in shopping and money-handling skills, and enjoyed doing some cooking. She quickly learnt to fill her pill box independently, and took her medication regularly.

As the centre was short-staffed, a volunteer was organized to take Mary to her classes at the adult education centre, as well as give Mary extra attention in class or help her to socialize with other class members. To give her some practice at using public transport, the volunteer also returned home with Mary on a bus on the two afternoons she had classes, rather than take the centre bus.

However, in the course of a four-month period, Mary became increasingly anxious on excursions out of the house, was refusing to go to the ATC or adult education classes and appeared to be losing weight. The consultant psychiatrist continued to monitor the situation.

During this time, an electrical fault in the refrigerator caused a fire in the flat, which led to complete destruction of its interior. The two women escaped, although Mary sustained burns to her hands which led to her hospitalization in a general hospital ward for two weeks. The nurses described her as a 'model' patient – bright, cheery and interested in what was happening on the ward. The OT and social worker noticed this also, in contrast to her agitation prior to the fire in the house.

The dramatic change of attitude confirmed once more the impact of isolation and limited peer contact in contributing to Mary's distress and agitation. There were still no vacancies in the local hostel, and Mary remained in hospital for a further 2 weeks.

Whilst emergency accommodation was being organized by the social worker, the OT continued to visit Mary weekly.

Mary and her mother moved to their new home 4 weeks after the fire and programmes as outlined previously continued, in addition to a visit to the library once a week. She seemed to enjoy this very much, and often used the opportunity to go to the shops. At this time, all those involved in supporting Mary and her mother met to clarify tasks and aims.

However, in the course of three months she again deteriorated, was losing weight, refusing to go out, shrieking at her mother and was rehospitalized.

Readmission and discharge After four weeks in hospital, Mary was discharged home. She was adamant that she would not go back to the ATC. A referral to a psychiatric day centre was rejected on the grounds that she would 'not cope', even though many of the organized activities, such as crafts and cooking, were ones she could participate in. The social worker worked on looking for other suitable day centres, as well as pressuring the hostel to consider Mary's urgent need for accommodation.

Mary no longer went to the ATC or classes, although the ATC agreed to leave Mary's place open for a few months.

The twice-weekly visits continued, concentrating on shopping, going to the library, and encouraging Mary in her reading and knitting.

About two months after her return, Mary's mother and sister-in-law reported that Mary had been soiling her clothes and bed and that she kept saying she didn't have a head/body. Mary was very agitated and distractible, shouted at others, and ate poorly. Contact with the psychiatrist to inform her of Mary's deterioration led to readmission for one month.

Subsequent discharge lasted one month, when Mary was again readmitted in a very distressed state, and doubly incontinent. The hostel was pressed by the social worker and OT to accommodate Mary, to which they agreed, and a gradual programme to introduce Mary to the hostel was organized. (Over a three-week period she had several meals there and slept there overnight.)

The OT passed on relevant information to the hostel staff about Mary's skills and interests, as well as some of her difficulties. After Mary moved to the hostel, the OT visited several times before ceasing her visits. Discussions during this time centred around the difference between the hostel and her home, and the fact that the OT would no longer be visiting her. OT intervention was no longer needed as the care workers there were able to give Mary the direction she needed in order to develop independence skills and give her the support she needed.

OT intervention with this client over an 18-month period, involved the OT in:

1. Enabling independence in ADL skills;
2. Devising opportunities for Mary to get out of the house;
3. Regular liaison with other workers involved in supporting Mary, particularly the psychiatrist and hospital staff;
4. Being a social contact for Mary.

SOME PROBLEMS AND THEIR ALLEVIATION

Turnover of carers

Despite community and government support, fuelled with normalization philosophy and a more positive outlook for people with mental handicaps living in the community, a high rate of care worker stress and staff turnover has been observed (McCord, 1981).

The reluctant loss of expertise, lowering of morale and change of staff can be distressing for clients, and their families, as well as being disruptive to any programmes being implemented, particularly for more disabled clients. Time out, peer group support and supervision may provide some relief although respite care and staff training might also be indicated.

Respite Care

There is a strong case for using short-term care facilities for clients with demanding or antisocial behaviours living in staffed houses. This may seem a contradiction in terms, that paid staff in a supportive housing scheme would appear to need a 'break' from one of the residents. However, people living and working in a small group home take on the semblance of a family. The use and importance of respite care for families (or foster families) caring for a family member who is mentally handicapped is well recognized (Bruininks *et al.*, 1980; Gathercole, 1981a; Paterson, 1986; Shearer, 1986).

Just as families feel the need for a 'break' from a disturbed or demanding family member, so do other residents and staff in a group home. It may be a vital resource in maintaining the energy and enthusiasm of staff in a stressful work situation, as well as protecting others living in the house from extreme behaviours.

Staff training

The need for on-going staff training is even more important for carers working with more handicapped individuals. Whilst the organization of such training is very much the province of managers, the OT needs to emphasize to staff working with this very disabled group of clients:

1. The importance of structuring the day (as in 24-hour planning);
2. The types of activities that can be used to stimulate profoundly handicapped individuals (see OT Approaches);
3. Structuring the environment and the activity itself (i.e. minimizing the distractions in an area where an activity is taking place, breaking the activity down into its component parts – see Chapter 4).

Client distress and illness

The incidence of mental illness and behaviour disturbances amongst people with mental handicap would suggest the obvious need for access and availability to psychiatric care in the community setting. There is some dispute whether this would best be achieved by: (a) specialised psychiatric units for people with handicaps versus integration into mainstream services or (b) separate behaviour training units or more training in the home setting (McBrien, 1987), respectively. Without going into the politics of the matter, the availability of facilities for clients with behaviour or psychiatric problems is the key to their maintenance in the community.

The importance of identifying such needs in individuals prior to the move to a community house cannot be over-emphasized. Experience has shown that lack of attention to such details creates stressful situations for all those working with the individual concerned, be they care staff or occupational therapists.

Access to medical back-up in terms of physicians, ophthalmologists and dentists is vital to enable all people with mental handicaps to live in the community, particularly those who are very disabled (Bruininks et al., 1980; Kinnell, 1987). Although this is an obvious statement to make, experience has shown the importance of identifying and accessing such services, prior to the community move rather than have to expend time and energy afterward, which might infringe on therapeutic input into training programmes, leisure activities, etc. Kinnell outlines how general practitioners and medical specialists could improve their service provision to this client group.

Poor care practices

Limited ability to communicate, as well as physical dependence on others for their care, makes people with profound handicaps vulnerable to dubious care practices. The importance of evaluation and monitoring of staffed housing has been mentioned in Chapter 5, and this is even more the case when very disabled people are concerned.

SUMMARY

This chapter has focused on the particular needs of people with profound mental handicap, behaviour problems and mental illness and the contributions that the OT can make for such clients with regard to skill acquisition, integration into the community and development of interests. Other community resources needed to help maintain such disabled people in the community with a good quality of life have been identified.

Despite much political goodwill and more positive community support for de-institutionalization and setting up of community services for people with mental handicaps, the result of one study suggests that the community may lack the facilities to cater for the needs of people with profound handicaps (Best-Sigford et al., 1982). The authors found that one-half of the readmissions to institutions in the United States in the year of their study were people who were severely or profoundly handicapped.

In such dubious circumstances, it is essential that the resources needed for each individual are identified and organized prior to the move. If unavailable, it may be worth considering postponement of the move until the necessary resources can be mobilized.

7

Individual and group work

PSYCHODYNAMIC PROCESSES

Although there are many and varied definition and descriptions of psychotherapy and none universally agreed upon (Szymanski, 1980), it can be defined as a 'contracted' interpersonal relationship where one (the client) enters because of some emotional/interpersonal difficulty and the other (the therapist) helps the person to overcome this via special skills and training which he/she possesses. The relationship has a beginning and an end, with meetings at set times in set places. The term psychotherapy is often interchanged with 'guidance' or 'counselling'.

The basic aims of psychotherapy have been summed up by Malan (1979) as: (a) helping the client to gain insight into his/her maladaptive behaviour; (b) enable the client to face what he/she really feels and fears such that (c) real feelings may be utilized within relationships (and in various situations), thus changing maladaptive into adaptive behaviour. The effects of this 'emotional learning' should be permanent, such that the client should be able to deal with the situation at hand and similar ones in the future.

Psychotherapy takes place in individual, group and family contexts. Teaching clients to gain independence in tasks either individually or in a group setting involves psychodynamic processes. This chapter will primarily address the application of individual and group processes for adults with a mental handicap, and family approaches will be discussed in Chapter 9.

UNDERSTANDING DISTURBED BEHAVIOUR

Maladaptive or disturbed behaviour may have a wide variety of causes and sources. It can be useful to examine such behaviour in people with mental handicaps in light of their own perceptions of the world and personal experiences.

With particular regard to the severely handicapped, Spensley (1984) notes an emphasis in the UK of dealing with disturbed behaviour via behaviour modification, where 'sadness' is often confused with 'badness'. In the absence of the verbal skills to express himself and out of sheer frustration, a person may resort to extreme behaviour, such as destroying furniture. Spensley suggests that trying to understand the (disabled) person's perceptions of the world and context of behaviour, may be a more useful approach for carers/therapists to adopt when working with severely mentally handicapped people. That is not to say that analysis and understanding of the behaviour from the client's point of view will bring forth a magical solution. It can, however, enable the therapist to see things from the client's point of view, and from there, generate possible actions, some of which may not have been considered previously.

Mental handicap has also been considered as a 'defence' against trauma (Mannoni, 1973; Sinason, 1986), whereby the individual projects 'stupidness' or exaggerates physical disability (e.g. by slurring words or slumping in a chair) in order to protect his/herself from further painful experiences. In a similar vein, it has been suggested that powerful emotional factors may 'block' a person's ability to learn and perform daily living tasks, irrespective of identified mental handicap or not (Doll, 1953; Gunzberg, 1974). (Symington (1981), however, notes that it may not be that easy to distinguish 'organic' from emotional factors.)

These comments would seem to suggest that a psychotherapeutic approach to understanding and tackling maladaptive or disturbed behaviours might be usefully employed. This is of great relevance to occupational therapists or any other care workers in contact with handicapped clients with behavioural or emotional disturbances.

Disturbed behaviour may also be attributable to physical illness (Spencer, 1987), psychiatric disorder, or environmental change (e.g. transition shock after leaving an institution for the community, Coffman and Harris, 1980) which need to be checked and taken into account prior to the implementation of behavioural or psychodynamic type interventions.

PSYCHOTHERAPY AND MENTAL HANDICAP

Psychotherapy of mentally handicapped and non-handicapped persons is essentially similar in form and structure, although therapeutic goals and techniques will vary depending on the degree of disability, particularly in terms of communicative and cognitive skills (Szymanski, 1980). With people who have a mental handicap, psychotherapy can be expanded to include verbal and non-verbal techniques (e.g. art, play, action techniques) (Gunzberg, 1974; Selan, 1976; Szymanski, 1980; Matson, 1984). Stress is placed on the diversity of approaches that can be used (Monfils and Menolascino, 1984), which include hypnosis, and suggestions as to how individual therapy can be adapted for the client with mental handicap are also made (Halpern and Berard, 1974).

Eclectic approach

Clarke (1984) views the 'eclectic' approach to psychotherapy with people who have mental handicaps in terms of: (a) the setting in which therapy takes place; (b) the medium and techniques used, and (c) the theoretical standpoint of the therapist.

The setting chosen should depend on where: (a) the client appears to be able to communicate best (either verbally or non-verbally); (b) the behaviours to be modified are demonstrated; (c) variability of emotional and personal expression are enhanced, and (d) privacy quietness are provided. Technique of selection relates to the need and skills of the client (e.g. for stimulation or 'sedation' in terms of activity level) that will enable expression of feelings or thoughts. Similarly, Clarke notes that the 'theoretical standpoint' taken by the therapist, be it 'Rogerian', 'analytic' or other should again be modified according to what the client will respond to.

Maintaining a broad view and range of approaches certainly gives the therapist opportunity to respond to a variety of needs and situations. However, it also highlights the need for good supervision and training of the therapist for appropriate selection and implementation of method (see later).

An important premise underlying the use of such techniques with this client group is that mental handicap does not imply that the individual's emotional needs are 'handicapped' or any less than a non-handicapped person. This is well illustrated by bereavement work with mentally handicapped people who have lost their parents/

145

carers (Oswin, 1981; Kitching, 1987). People with mental handicaps also pass through the same 'stages' of mourning and present their grief in a variety of ways as do non-handicapped people (Oswin, 1981). What these authors both emphasize is that the handicapped person may need to work through their grief, with structured guidance – a variety of examples are given – to ensure they progress through the bereavement and come to terms with the loss, and that their grief is no less than that experienced by a non-handicapped relative.

Historical overview

The writings on the use of psychotherapeutic techniques (from the 1920s to the 1940s) with people who have a mental handicap are scarce (Clarke, 1984; Monfils and Menolascino, 1984). This can possibly be attributed to the fact that the psychotherapy techniques used at that time were mostly of a psychoanalytic nature. Beliefs were held that 'poor' verbal and lack of 'abstract-conceptual' skills would be barriers to gaining 'insight', and that the tendency to dependency would be an obstacle to the resolution of 'transference', which would undermine the therapy process (Szymanski, 1980). Other beliefs, such as: 'normal' cognitive skills are necessary for gaining insight: and that mentally handicapped people react to external reality only and are unable to perceive consequences or respond to others' needs; are noted as other reasons for excluding children and adults with mental handicap from psychotherapy (Syzmanski, Clarke).

More recent studies and case examples, however, describe an enthusiastic upswing in the successful use of psychotherapeutic techniques, both in the individual and group settings, which provide a clear picture of precesses and common themes. For those who wish to read further, see Astrachan, 1955; Slivkin and Bernstein, 1968; Baran, 1972; Mannoni, 1973; Heller, 1978; Symington, 1981; Spensley, 1984; Balbernie, 1985a,b; Hodgetts, 1986; McGowan, 1986; Sinason, 1986; Balbernie, 1987; Kitching, 1987; Cole, 1989).

Client Selection

The various criteria for identifying clients with mental handicap who might benefit from group or individual psychotherapy are very wide. Reference is made to IQ level, with Clarke (1984) identifying a score of 45–50 as being the lowest parameter for considering a person suitable for individual psychotherapy. (This reasoning is that clients with higher IQ score will inevitably have social and adjustment problems, i.e. maladaptive behaviour, which would make them good candidates for therapy, unlike those with lower 'scores', who have not even developed certain adaptive behaviours.) It is also considered that 'therapeutic' assistance should be made available, irrespective of IQ, to those who are motivated to change and demonstrate a degree of insight (Gunzberg, 1974; Monfils and Menolscino, 1984). Factors such as maladaptive behaviour, awareness of distress and desire to effect change, ability to respond to a warm supportive relationship, presence of mental disturbance in which psychological factors play an aetiological role, ability to communicate to some degree verbally or non-verbally, and the expectation that the amelioration or psychological symptoms will improve a person's ability to use his cognitive potential are further indications for suitability for psychotherapy (Gunzberg, 1974; Szymanski, 1980; Matson, 1984; Monfils and Menolascino, 1984).

The ability to communicate and feel comfortable in a group is a clear determinant of selecting individual or group therapy (Clarke). Physical or sensory defects need not rule out some clients as candidates, but merely determine the nature of the therapy used (Clarke), or equipment needed (Crawford, 1987). Szymanski emphasizes the importance of psychotherapy taking place in the context of other therapeutic, educational and habilitative goals and may indicate the need for contact with the family and other care workers, but without disturbing the confidentiality aspect of the therapeutic relationship (see later).

Therapist variables

As well as the client presenting certain attributes and behaviour which would indicate his/her need and suitability for therapy, the therapist must be able to identify if he/she has the skills required to do the job.

Important skills for therapists working in groups or individually with this client group, in a psychotherapeutic way, include: (a) a positive attitude to mental handicap and acceptance of the client, given his/her limitations; (b) knowledge about the medical aspects of mental handicap (e.g. genetics, epilepsy, commonly used anticonvulsants), personality theory and abnormal (and normal) human

Table 7.1 Problems in rehabilitation of adults with a mental handicap, living in the community. N = 97; females = 43, males = 54. Age range - 16 to 65 years; median age = 21 years

Problem dealt with in psychotherapy	No. of Ss (N = 97)
Personal and interpersonal problems	36
Difficulties in locating suitable jobs	25
Difficulties due to other disabilities, mostly physical	21
Upsetting family problems	19
Slowness in leaving job	19
Insufficient vocational training or job experience	7
Previous job failures caused employer resistance	7
Other problems (e.g. poor health, requested job very close to home)	5

development; (c) patience and ability to tolerate frustration, either in terms of slow progress towards goals or struggle of clients to express themselves; (d) warmth, empathy and be able to maintain the necessary commitment to the client, and (e) knowledge of other community services in order to maintain a broad perspective in terms of service availability and services used by the client (Monfils and Menolascino, 1984).

Although the authors make special reference to skills needed by therapists working in a psychotherapeutic mode, they are attributes with which any therapist working with this client group should identify.

Themes

Of interest to therapists working with adults with a mental handicap in the community is the study by Di Michael and Terwillinger (1953) who followed up 97 mentally handicapped subjects with a variety of physical disabilities, living in the community, in different parts of the USA who had received some form of counselling or psychotherapy. Table 7.1 summarizes their findings which list the problems that were dealt with psychotherapeutically.

Other themes noted to emerge in individual and group psychotherapy with people with a mental handicap (Szymanski and Rosefsky, 1980; Monfils and Menolascino, 1984) are summarized in Table 7.2.

Adding to these lists could include the movement out of institution to community, a situation which Matson (1984) believes will generate a further need for psychotherapeutic intervention.

Table 7.2 Emergent themes in group and individual psychotherapy with people who have a mental handicap

Individual and group (Monfils and Menolascino, 1984)	Group (Szymanski and Rosefsky, 1980)
Inadequate self-image	Independence and future plans
Sexual problems (knowledge, premarital counselling, contraception)	Dealing with being handicapped
Interpersonal relationships	Appropriate social behaviour
Understanding emotions, channelling feelings appropriately	Relating to peers
Feelings about being handicapped	Expression of feelings
Separation from family	
Moving out of home, into community residence	
Transition from school to vocational placement	

Goals and objectives

For therapy to be effective, goals and objectives must be set at the very beginning and be clearly defined (Szymanski, 1980; Monfils and Menolascino, 1984); this is particularly important for the client with a mental handicap. He/she must understand the reason for referral into therapy; a contract, be it verbal or written, between the client and therapist may be a useful tool in goal setting (Monfils and Menolascino).

Some commonly encountered goals of psychotherapy include helping the individual to understand his strengths, setting realistic expectations, improving impulse control and frustration tolerance, recognizing and expressing emotions appropriately and overcoming egocentricity (Szymanski). Monfils and Menolascino note the importance of determining short-term as against long-term goals, to ensure this coincides with the number of sessions and time available to both therapist and client.

Other goals of psychotherapy noted by Clarke include the creation of 'cathartic' and 'sedative' influences, with regard to the way the individual deals with situations, or 'didactic', as in teaching the client new ways of tackling difficulties.

Some basic objectives for therapists/counsellors involved in working with people with mental handicaps have been defined by Thorne (1948) to include: (1) accepting the individual as being a worthwhile person despite his disabilities; (2) permitting expression and clarification of emotional reactions; (3) teaching methods for resisting frustration, and achieving emotional control; (4) outlining standards of acceptable conduct within the ability of each individual; (5) building up self-confidence and respect by providing experiences of success, and (6) training the individual to seek help through the counselling process.

What follows is a more detailed discussion of processes, dynamics and techniques used in individual and group work. They have been divided up to provide clarity, although in reality there is much overlap between the two, and issues which arise in both settings.

INDIVIDUAL WORK

Individual psychotherapy will be viewed in terms of techniques used, stages of therapy, themes emerging, therapist variables to note, family contact, and other issues, such as transference and resistance, which are common in psychotherapy with the non-handicapped population. Assessing suitability for therapy has been dealt with in the previous section.

Techniques

Directiveness

Both Szymanski and Monfils and Menolascino emphasize the importance of directiveness in therapy with people who have a mental handicap. Brief psychotherapy and behaviour therapy are examples of more directive approaches (Szymanski).

Directiveness does not imply quashing the client's feelings or expression, but refers to limit setting as to what is acceptable or unacceptable behaviour. There is little to be gained from allowing a person to sleep through a session or to destroy the room in which sessions take place. Poor personal boundary definition or not knowing how to act in a given situation, emphasizes the importance of the therapist being very directive in therapy sessions (Szymanski).

Limits can be set in clear, brief concrete form without criticism, e.g. 'We must behave quietly in order not to disturb others in the clinic', as against 'Do not make so much noise' (Szymanski). In the case of inappropriate behaviours being the result of excessive stimulation, Szymanski suggests that desensitization may be used, i.e. first talking about the situation (e.g. visit to a cafe), then role playing (e.g. going to the cafe, ordering a drink) and later taking increasingly longer trips/visits (e.g. to the cafe).

Within the limits set, the therapist can give the individual opportunity for spontaneous expression, and appropriate feedback. The
therapist should not force an issue or use leading questions but
should indirectly lead the individual in the desired direction by use
of limit setting (Szymanski), and appropriate choice of therapy
techniques.

Verbal techniques

The words and expressions used with this kind of client should be
brief, concrete, clear and suited to the individual's level of language
development and comprehension (Szymanski; Monfils and Menolascino). Metaphors and expressions within cultural context may need
to be used (see case study later) or communication devices
(Crawford, 1987), e.g. word processor, use of Makaton signs,
pictures, etc. If using verbal techniques, much will be gained from
dealing with issues in the 'here and now', with the use of concrete
illustrations of the client's behaviour (Szymanski); many people with
a mental handicap find exploration of the past and projection into the
future difficult, and report views that are either unreliable, irrelevant
or completely unrealistic.

Dwelling on interesting fantasy material and long periods of
silence should be avoided (Szymanski). Time spent examining the
fantasies of clients with a mental handicap can weaken the
individual's ability to test reality, and distances him/her from the
'here and now' dealings of their particular difficulty. Silences
generally occur with this client group not because of resistance but
because he/she does not know what to say, and based on past
experiences of ridicule, the person is fearful of saying something
wrong. At times silence may reflect anxiety about a particular issue,
in which case warm support by the therapist is usually sufficient to
overcome it. Generally speaking, a silent, staring therapist is seen as
rejecting and critical by this client group.

Non-verbal techniques

There is much written about the use of play therapy as a medium
for work with children who have a mental handicap or other
emotional disturbance (Axline, 1969; Gunzberg, 1974; Kelly, 1981;
Matson, 1984; Balbernie, 1987). A wide variety of equipment is
described ranging from toys and art equipment (e.g. Axline; Balbernie) to specific use of puppets (e.g. Kelly).

151

Although perhaps not seen as 'age-appropriate' in normalization terms, the use of some of this media may be particularly useful for clients with less developed verbal skills and who express themselves well through the production of items, e.g. through paint or clay. Puppetry has indeed been used successfully in programmes with adults who have a mental handicap to improve communication skills, teach sex education and for assertiveness training (Page, 1986).

The use of media requires the therapist to be comfortable both in terms of skill needed to use the material, and deciding on the best way to use it, e.g. asking the person to do a painting of his family. Selecting and identifying the media that the client will best respond to requires thought and consideration. Again these concerns point to the necessity of the therapist to receive supervision.

Other non-verbal techniques include modelling, behaviour rehearsal, relaxation and desensitization procedures (Monfils and Menolascino). These authors view behavioural techniques involving a good deal of structure to be most appropriate in teaching adaptive behaviour to more severely and profoundly handicapped people.

In working with a client with a psychosis, Monfils and Menolascino emphasize the value of giving the individual feedback through body posture, facial expression, or verbal content about the immediate environment. From an OT viewpoint, this may be hard to achieve through a more verbally orientated approach, and better dealt with through activities of meaning to the client. The 'degree' of psychotic activity, preoccupation with 'voices' and level of disturbance, will of course affect the degree to which the individual is accessible to any kind of human contact or activity.

Other factors which may aid the therapist include the setting up of the room and proximity to the client (see Chapter 4). 'Tuning in' to any idiosyncratic expressions or behaviours of clients can be helpful in anticipating client distress and relevant therapist action (Szymanski). For example, 'Mary' (referred to in Chapter 6) would show her distress by saying very loudly 'I haven't got a head, I haven't got a body.' By this, the OT working with Mary was able to see she was in some distress, identify possible causes for it (e.g. an upset with her sister-in-law, worries about her future, etc.) and modify the tasks she would get Mary to do.

Lastly, Szymanski notes that video taping sessions may help the therapist to examine non-verbal communications more closely, and identify appropriate responses.

Stages of therapy

The process of psychotherapy is commonly divided into three stages: initial, middle and termination (Szymanski). (This is not unlike the processes for group/team work and therapy, i.e. forming, warming, storming, norming, conforming and adjourning – see Chapter 1.) The stages are not sharply delineated and the individual may move forward and back through the stages depending on the topic at hand or external events which may disturb him/her. Szymanski notes that although certain themes may be typical for certain stages, they may recur, given that people with a mental handicap have a tendency to regress and a need for repetition.

Initial phase

The initial phase is characterized by setting the 'ground rules' and clarifying the reasons for therapy as well as establishing an alliance and rapport with the client (Szymanski, 1980; Monfils and Menolascino, 1984; Menolascino, Gilson and Levitas, 1986).

Ground rules refers to time, place and length of sessions, and what is deemed acceptable and unacceptable behaviour, although this may arise during the course of therapy. What is very important is that the therapist is clear in his/her mind as to what limits on behaviour are to be set from the beginning, and to be prepared to act at any time if/when the situation arises.

Clarifying the reasons for therapy is important for both client and therapist. The therapist must ensure that the client understands why he/she is there; it may be useful to establish a verbal or written contract in order to establish the boundaries and goals of sessions (Monfils and Menolascino). The problems and situations that have led the client into therapy can be discussed, given the language and cognitive skills of the client (Szymanski). This should be done in clear and concrete terms, without criticism or blame. For example, 'Your parents would like you to be happier' is far better than 'Your mother has complained that you hit her.' Szymanski also notes that putting the problem in a 'collaborative' form can sometimes be appealing. For example, 'Your problem is that you get angry and say things too fast; many people have the same trouble. You and I are going to learn to fight this problem.'

It is unrealistic to assume that all clients presenting to the therapist will be suitable for therapy. It is very important that some of the criteria mentioned earlier are apparent upon referral and for the therapist to receive/gather sufficient information beforehand. For example, the therapist needs to be sure that there is no serious medical or florid mental illness which might be contributing to the client's disturbances, and of other agencies/care personnel working with the client. It may be necessary to clarify the situation on the basis of an assessment interview, which is a frequently used procedure (Malan, 1979), in which case it is important that the client and the referring agency (if any) understand this to be the case.

The therapist must work swiftly in the initial phase to establish an 'alliance' with the client (Menolascino, Gilson and Levitas). This is particularly important as, generally speaking, people with mental handicaps do not have the same opportunities as others to make major decisions about their lives and exercise control. The essence of therapy is to build up self-esteem and mastery over a situation; the fact that the therapist is seen as an 'enabler', via an alliance in which both therapist and client participate, is the key to the success of therapy. The client needs to see that the therapist communicates to him in a 'language' he understands, and is interested and concerned.

Middle phase

Having established an 'alliance' and rapport, the bulk of psycho-therapeutic work can take place, as it does, in this stage. Szymanski indicates some specific actions for therapists during this stage to enable the client to 'reveal' and 'explore' his/her particular situation and difficulties. These include:

1. Using him/herself as a therapeutic tool, e.g. by serving as a model for the client to identify with by talking about or demonstrating how he would act in situations similar to those under discussion;
2. Being supportive to the client, but encouraging him/her also to be 'self-supporting' by reinforcing his/her strengths and avoiding dependency as much as possible;
3. Enabling the client to understand his/her situation, by organizing observations of the client in a clear and concrete form, and presenting them to him/her in a 'language' that is understood;
4. Discussing issues relating to the client's difficulties in order for the client to gain some understanding into the situation; confrontations should be avoided (e.g. 'Tell me how you feel about being handicapped'), and instead, the client 'led' to bring it up on

his/her own (e.g. 'You told me you have been called names by other people. It's unfair and must be difficult on you. What names did they call you?');

5. The therapist must be clear about what the client means by using certain terms. For example, if the client mentions he is 'handicapped' or 'slow', the therapist should explore what the client means by this term. It may be necessary for the therapist to give an explanation of what the term means, and should do so by using descriptive and non-derogative terms, e.g. if a person has a mental handicap, he has 'troubles in learning'. Support and empathy are useful tools to employ in painful situations, such as this, e.g. Therapist: 'I can't read music – it's a sort of mental handicap in music.'

Szymanski concludes by saying that the goal of this phase of therapy is for the client to be able to transfer insight and knowledge gained into constructive behaviours and approaches to his/her situation.

Termination phase

Termination is generally difficult and a threatening phase for most people engaged in psychotherapy (Malan, 1979), more for those who have a mental handicap, because of the tendency to dependence and sensitivity to rejection (Szymanski).

The impending termination of therapy may evoke regression, depression and acting out (Szymanski). This indicates that the preparation for termination should be gradual and done throughout therapy. Vacations and other absences of the therapist can be usefully employed as starting points for analysing the client's reaction to past losses and preparing for the loss of the therapist. Having a set 'timetable' either for the duration of therapy (e.g. if it is for a set number of sessions) or a 'countdown' to the last session can be useful. Issues such as the client's perception of the termination and any associated feelings (e.g. anger) should be explored either verbally or through 'play'.

Although Szymanski has made these comments in terms of people with mental handicap, many of the features of termination mentioned also emerge in therapy with non-handicapped clients (see case examples of Malan) and in group work (Crawley, 1979).

155

Contact with the family

For clients living with relatives, casework with the family is an important part of the psychotherapy process, because they are people the client interacts with (Szymanski). As with learning to implement other daily living skills, the home environment must be encouraging and accepting for practice to take place. It is therefore very important for the therapist to inform and enable those living with the client to allow him/her to 'exercise' new skills learnt in psychotherapy. For those clients living in a staffed group home, it is likely that the therapist will need to communicate to care staff in some form also.

Guidelines for communicating and working with close relatives of clients engaged in psychotherapy are noted by Szymanski. These include:

1. The parents are not 'in therapy' nor should they be treated as the needy clients;
2. Caution should be exercised not to aggravate any feelings of guilt, for their child's handicap or maladjustment;
3. The therapist should present explicitly and clearly to the parents the relevance of the therapy to their child in concrete terms; for example, the goals of identifying and then teaching appropriate behaviour management techniques to parents is more acceptable and specific than 'helping with feelings about the child';
4. Parents may be seen jointly, with the client participating for part of the session – in this way the therapist can observe the relative – client interactions. This may be a time when parents can use the therapist as a model for communicating with the relative, setting limits, expectations and giving support. It may also be useful to include siblings in such meetings. (See the next chapter for more details on family work.)

Some of the topics noted by Szymanski that can emerge with contact with parents/relatives of clients engaged in psychotherapy are summarized in Table 7.3.

Other Issues

Aside from dealing with the specific difficulty that the client presents with, other issues may emerge in the therapy process. These factors, commonly emerging in psychotherapy with non-handicapped people

Table 7.3 Issues encountered with parents/relatives of clients who have a mental handicap and are engaged in psychotherapy

Parent education	Emotional adjustment	Family adjustment
1. Behaviour management techniques	1. Adaptation to child's handicap and dealing with associated feelings, e.g. guilt depression, anger	1. Marital conflict particularly regarding the handicapped relative
2. Specific developmental delays, abilities, needs of relative	2. Own needs for emotional fulfilment, privacy	2. Needs of siblings
3. Techniques to aid independence skills of relative	3. Learning to achieve gratification from the child	3. Handicapped person's role in family dynamics
4. Future planning for 'normalized' living		
5. Sex education		
6. Resource finding		

also, may hinder the progress of therapy. They are identified here to alert therapists to their presence, and may come into play in 'non-verbal' (e.g. play, action method, art-orientated) work also.

Transference

Transference refers to the development of intense feelings for the therapist by the client; frequently, these feeling belong to someone in the client's past and have been transferred to the therapist (Malan, 1979).

In order to use the transference to therapeutic gain, the therapist must be able to:

1. Recognize and accept the transference;
2. Interpret it to the client;
3. Perceive the way it originated; and
4. Interpret this to the client too (Malan).

Transference is a means by which the therapist can utilize feelings buried in the client's past, that have emerged in sessions, to explore and hopefully resolve them, and enable the client to deal with similar situations more constructively in the future.

In relation to clients with a mental handicap in therapy, Szymanski notes that the form of the transference can differ from the non-handicapped population. He attributes this to: (a) a tendency to regression; (b) fear of anything that might sound like criticism or rejection from the therapist; and (c) fear of the therapist finding out about his/her shortcomings or behaving inappropriately. He notes that regression may be a form of expressing anger.

A good example of transference in non-verbal therapy work is described by Thomas and Howard (1971) who write about their input with a severely handicapped young man, who self-mutilated; they used water-based activities as a part of therapy. After returning from holiday, the therapist was rebuffed by the young man, who spoke for the first time in years, claiming that he felt abandoned, indicating the transfer of feelings of dependency to the therapist.

Lastly, Malan notes that in order to handle transferences, the therapist needs to be reasonably secure and insightful in themselves. Supervision is also an important tool that can help the therapist to understand transferences received and use them for therapeutic gain.

Resistance

Resistance in psychotherapy refers to the 'fight' the client puts up against becoming aware of painful feelings (Malan). Various actions may be used to achieve this, e.g. changing the subject, denial, projections on to the therapist, coming late or missing appointments. Silence in sessions is often interpreted as resistance (Malan, although this may not necessarily be the case with regard to clients who have a mental handicap, where silence generally has more to do with not knowing what to say and fear of saying the wrong thing (Szymanski).

Malan noes that resistance may occur if the therapist 'gets ahead' of the client's emotional capacity, or it may be part of a transference. For example, the client may be anxious about trusting the therapist because his/her trust has been misplaced by another person in the past – this feeling is thus transferred to the therapist. Resistance can be dealt with by using further interpretations or by changing the therapy mode, e.g. from verbal to action method (Malan).

With regard to clients with a mental handicap, Szymanski suggests that resistance occurs less often, because of 'lack of defences' and 'high dependency needs'. Parental resistance can also be a block to the therapy of their child (Mannoni, 1973), taking the form of ignoring the child's progress, withdrawal from therapy or presenting to the therapist their own problems (see Mannoni p. 81–91 for case study illustrations).

Countertransference

Countertransference refers to transference directed back to the client (in therapy) from the therapist; it is the response of the therapist to the transference (feelings and emotions) directed to his/her from the client.

Countertransference can lead the therapist into a variety of precarious situations, both with the client or his family, which can 'disturb' the therapy process Szymanski includes the following situations where:

1. The therapist has a wish to 'cure' the client, directing the client into harbouring unrealistic expectations and achieving behaviour changes that are superficial, with the 'core' symptoms being suppressed;
2. The therapist with 'rescue wishes' who tends to identify and over-protect the client, thereby encouraging 'acting-out', and
3. The therapist is drawn into play the 'adoptive parent', finding him/herself in competition with the client's (child's) parents.

These countertransference situations further emphasize the need for good training and case supervision (Szymanski), so that the therapist can look at his/her work from an objective distance and plan suitable therapeutic responses. (See later in the chapter for further discussion.)

Anxiety

Anxiety can be viewed as a symptom, not a behaviour, that can bring a person into therapy, and is frequently linked to some incident in the past (Malan). In relation to individual therapy with clients who have a mental handicap, Mannoni notes anxiety to be particularly related to: (1) establishing communication with the therapist; once this is achieved, anxiety diminishes; (2) fears of parents/primary care givers with regard to therapy; this can sometimes 'pressure' the therapist in terminating therapy early, leaving the client with problems unresolved; (3) the fear of a 'cure', e.g. how will the parents/family adjust to have a 'more competent' person in their midst and how will the client feel about dealing competently with previously difficult situations? This is connected with ideas of using mental handicap as a defence against trauma (Mannoni, 1973; Sinason, 1986), where the client must risk being 'unmasked' and

159

exposing their competence and potential, and (4) the realization of caregivers that a magical 'cure' cannot be evoked.

Confidentiality

Confidentiality of sessions with the client is essential in order to establish trust and enable the client to 'reveal' his/herself (Szymanski 1980; Balbernie, 1987). Doubtless other workers and/or family members may be curious to know what has been going on in therapy. Given the situation, it may be necessary to give these parties some 'message' about how the client is progressing in order for him/her to be able to 'practice' some of the skills learnt in sessions. This should only be done, however, with prior knowledge of the client and perhaps in his/her presence, if appropriate. This is illustrated in the following case study.

Case example

The following case example is included to illustrate many of the points made so far in this section on individual work. It highlights the emotional breadth of a person with a moderate degree of mental handicap and outwardly very immature, egocentric behaviour, and the need to use action and objects, as well as words in order to express ideas. Defence mechanisms, transference, counter-transference and interpretations are used, in conjunction with the imparting of basic information on some topics (e.g. death). Moreover, it shows that a person with a mental handicap can benefit from such individual work, that the therapist must have supervision, and that it is an area of work that OTs can tackle.

1. Client description and family

Hussein M., a young man of 20 years, of Turkish – Cypriot origin and Muslim faith was identified as having a mental handicap at an early age. He lived at home with his parents, sister Pina (29), and brother Nihat (17), with whom he shared a bedroom, in a three-bedroom, two-storey council flat on a quiet estate in South London. Another sister, Tula (27) lived nearby with her husband and family. Both Hussein and Pina had similar orofacial difficulties (a very complex cleft palate) in addition to mental handicap, and petit mal epilepsy. The family was tightly knit, had a small but supportive network of friends, but were very much on the periphery of the

Turkish community. They had emigrated to London largely because they hoped that Pina and Hussein could receive good medical attention.

Hussein attended a 2-year post-school programme in a local college, where emphasis was placed on developing living, social and leisure skills, and vocational options. At the time therapy intervention took place, Hussein had completed the second year of the course and was awaiting day centre placement, at an activity therapy centre (ATC) that Pina was currently attending.

2. *Reason for referral*

Hussein had been referred to the occupational therapist for home follow-up after he left school at 18 years. The OT worked with Hussein to transfer skills he had been learning at school (and subsequently college) to the home situation, and to assess his vocational potential. This took place over an 18-month period, by which the OT felt that she had achieved her initial aims.

However, over a two-month period, a series of incidents occurred: (1) The social worker, who gave Mr and Mrs M. a lot of support and organized the family's social security entitlements, left the district; (2) Hussein was unable to secure a place in the local day centre with a sheltered workshop, due to a shortage of places at the centre; (3) Mr M. was retrenched from his job, and six weeks later suffered a heart attack which left him with severe angina and a very poor prognosis; (4) Hussein was reported to be aggressive and threatening to his parents and fellow students at college; he was also picked up by a security guard for wandering around a Ministry of Defence establishment on three occasions, and had also been spotted standing in the middle of a major road 'conducting' the traffic. It was apparent that Hussein was reacting to this distressing set of circumstances. The OT decided that in addition to taking action in terms of situations (1) and (2), (writing letters to relevant agencies, agitating for a placement for Hussein, etc.), Hussein probably needed some time to talk about these events. In view of the fact that the OT would be leaving her job too within a three-month period, she decided to arrange to meet Hussein six times to: (a) find out if he understood what his father's illness entailed and that he might die; (b) assess the need for such meetings over a longer period of time; and (c) terminate the OTs relationship with him.

3. Meetings

Six meetings were organized to take place at college – Hussein had been allowed to stay on for an extra term. A quiet room next to the library was booked for these meetings and took place at a time when students were working on special projects; this had not been set up for Hussein, because he was only staying at college for one term.

4. General themes emerging in sessions

a. *Father's illness* – Hussein seemed to have little concept of his father's frailty or illness. Observing the scar left after the angiogram (Session 3) helped him to progress somewhat in his understanding with regard to the seriousness of the illness, although (by Session 5) he still clung on the vain hope that a dramatic recovery could be made. Some progress was made in terms of the reasons for the illness – from blaming his brother-in-law (Session 1) to blaming himself (Sessions 3 and 4). Further work would be needed to shift the 'cause' further, e.g. stress, worries, aging, etc.

b. *Death* – this subject was difficult for Hussein to broach in more than a superficial way (e.g. he stated that his father's death would mean that relatives from Cyprus would come to stay with the family for a while – Session 1.) He progressed to asking specific questions (would his father go to heaven – Session 3) and realization of his impotence in bringing people back to life – he was not able to bring his grandparents, who had died within the last few years, back to life (Session 5). More work was needed to be done on this area as Hussein was only partly able to look at death in relation to his father, and perhaps needed more specific information about burial, etc.

c. *Control* – this progressed from Hussein projecting himself as omnipotent (e.g. able to organize a job for his father, Sessions 1,2) to being able to recognize the situations he could and couldn't control. For example, he could make Christmas decorations and keep his 'good' self in control but could not stop people coming in and out of the family home, which disturbed his routine, or make his grandparents come back from the dead – Session 5. He was learning to modify his responses to situations and approach them more realistically (e.g. could not cure father but could care for him, make him smile with a 'lion' flower – Session 3). His inability to assert himself in a constructive way at home and lack of control with regard to Mr M.'s illness (and prognosis) were areas that continued to thwart him.

d. *Defensive manoeuvres* – Although able to express emotion and feeling, Hussein employed a variety of defences which the OT had to combat. Examples include blaming his brother-in-law for Mr M.'s illness (Session 2), and changing the subject (Session 5). These manoeuvres were employed when the OT touched on sensitive issues, such as how he best support his father at home (Session 2).

e. *Adult or child* – Hussein moved between these two 'states' during all sessions, except for the fourth, when he was able to maintain adult composure throughout. He was ambivalent about becoming an adult and being forced to recognize his limitations, versus remaining protected and closeted from the world. (e.g. recognizing what he could/could not control versus wanting to know about games played at the day centre – Session 5).

f. *Good or bad* – Hussein recognized that he has an angel 'part' of him and a devil part, in Session 3:

> 'Hussein went into a long dialogue involving the Devil (who tells him to do bad things), Allah (from whom he asks forgiveness) and the Meluch (Angel, who will help him ''be good''). Hussein apologized to Allah for being bad and ''took'' the Devil out of his head (holding the Devil in his right fist). Feeling quite worried that Hussein would hold on to the Devil for ever, the OT suggested that the Devil had been very bad and began to ''jump'' on the floor. Hussein joined in too, dropped the Devil on the floor, picked him up and berated him verbally for being so wicked. Hussein decided that he would put the Devil in a cage at home, with a little bed, table and food. When challenged as to what he would do if the Devil whispered to him, Hussein said he would put the Meluch (Angel) in his head (which he then did with his left fist) who would tell him to be good.'

Here, Hussein recognizes that good and bad can exist in one person, and controls are required to keep the latter under control. He also demonstrates that he does not want to 'stamp out' the Devil completely, and in many ways deals with him quite fairly – with physical comforts!

g. *Actions and objects* – These prove useful in helping Hussein to express certain issues and highlight them for the therapist's attention (e.g. actions with Allah, Meluch and Devil (Session 3), Christmas decorations (Session 5).

5. *Achievement of initial aims?*

a. The sessions did permit the OT to impart some basic information to Hussein about illness and death, although he was still struggling with the finality of it all, in relation to his father specifically.

b. Throughout the course of the sessions, other areas did emerge which required on-going individual work. This included ambivalence about being an adult, conflict between living in two cultures (e.g. speaking Turkish at home and English at college – Session 3), asserting himself in a constructive way at home, issues of control (e.g. unable to control death but able to control the Devil – Session 5), and examining his own limitations. This became the basis for a referral to the psychiatrist for continued psychotherapy/counselling.

c. The fourth session did allow the OT time to talk about her departure with Hussein with some privacy, but as this was amidst many other issues, it was difficult to assess how Hussein interpreted it.

6. *Issues for the therapist*

Although the initial aims were achieved, the OT found the sessions hard work, and considered whether issues could have been dealt with differently:

a. The OT should have gathered some information about Muslim beliefs in relation to death, and burial rights, so that comments could be made in a cultural context. It might have also been useful to use pictures (e.g. of burial, coffin, etc.), working through a suitable book with Hussein or getting him to draw pictures about death and burial.

b. The OT found it difficult to 'draw out' Hussein once he employed a defensive manoeuvre, which tended to be towards the end of the session.

c. The OT became anxious at the prospect of Hussein hanging on to the Devil (Session 3), and directed him to punish it, showing the way herself by jumping on the Devil. Perhaps she should have not leapt in with this countertransference and allowed Hussein to find his own solution. On the other hand, the therapist was concerned that Hussein should not leave the session seeing himself as the total cause for Mr M.'s illness. As it happened, Hussein did not progress from this position, and it was identified as an area for continued exploration in longer term therapy.

d. The family session, although intended to be low key and orientated towards termination of the relationship, should have been better planned with Hussein's agreement. The OT risked betraying Hussein's confidence in her comments to the rest of the family.

e. The OT suggested psychiatric follow-up on an on-going individual basis but handover was not organised. This could have taken the form of a joint interview and/or of informing Hussein of the details (e.g. who the new therapist would be, how contact would be made, etc.).

f. Comments (a)–(e) indicate the need for on-going supervision in order to tackle these issues and examine alternative forms of action that could have been taken.

GROUP WORK

Literature reviews by Monfils and Menolascino (1984) and Szymanski and Rosefsky (1980) reveal extensive use of group work with people who have a mental handicap, as far back as the 1940s. Techniques described include group discussion, the use of non-verbal approaches, psychodrama, role play, pantomime, film, and structured social skills groups. The groups described include a wide spectrum of the handicapped population (i.e. from profound to mild mental handicap), although earlier studies relate more to those that are less disabled. The extensive range of groups and techniques described would suggest that group work is a very useful tool that can be utilized by therapists working with people who have a mental handicap, provided that they are open to using a variety of techniques, depending on clients' skills and needs. People with mental handicaps have been found to help each other learn in the pair or group setting (Wagner and Sternlicht, 1975; Favell, Favell and McGinsey, 1978; Storm and Willis, 1978).

It is worth noting that the same group processes and struggles emerge in group work as they do do with any other group. Reference has previously been made in Chapter 1 with regard to the group life cycle and formation/workings of multidisciplinary teams.

Whilst progressing through the cycle (forming, storming, norming, performing and adjourning – Crawley, 1978), group members will say certain things and demonstrate certain behaviours; the client with a mental handicap will do so likewise, but perhaps with more emphasis on non-verbal means of communication. Szymanski and

165

Table 7.4 Comparison of processes and therapist tasks in group life cycle (Crawley, 1979; Szymanski and Rosefsky, 1980)

Phase of group development	Likely patterns of group behaviour	Tasks for therapist
Forming	Dependence on leader; politeness; uncertainty about what to do; searching for sense of director (C) Why are we here? (S and R)	Guidance for members to feel 'safe'; freedom to let members start to take initiative (C) Specific guidance on group's purpose; getting people to introduce themselves formally, clearly establish ground rules (S and R)
Storming	Rebellion against leader; other members; sense of apathy, drifting hopelessness (C) Evaluation of leader, each other; power struggle between members; vieing for attention from leader; making fun of others, leader; challenging purposed group; ambivalence as group discussions not always about 'safe' issues (S and R)	Generate sense of security, that leader is strong, competent but not inflexible (C) Therapist directs group towards mutual support; restatement of members' problems in more detail (S and R)
Norming and performing	New sense of enthusiasm, trying out new ways of working; members taking more responsibility for group; group getting on with this job (C) Functioning as cohesive unit; expectation; giving of mutual support between members; recounting of problems; social meetings outside of group time; regressions to previous phases; attempts at independence (S and R)	Modelling of appropriate behaviour by leader; shaping of member responses; clarification of boundaries and rules; encouraging emergent leadership resources of group (C) Dealing with regressive behaviour (i.e. of earlier stage) (S and R)
Adjourning	Denial of end of group; regression to earlier stages; reminiscing about group; planning ending ceremony, revisions (C) Regression; planning future social meetings; apprehension at loss of group	Helping group to face up to ending and individuals to make future plans (C) Helping people to deal with loss of group; practice of difficult social situations that may be encountered via role play, practice

Table 7.5 Therapeutic factors in group psychotherapy (Yalom, 1975)

Factor	Description
Altruism	Helping others in the group and consequent increase in self-esteem, instead of feeling a 'burden
Cohesiveness	Feeling of togetherness of group members, of acceptance and reduced isolation from others
Universality	Perception that other group members have similar problems, feelings
Interpersonal learning	Learning about oneself and problems through feedback from others; practising different ways to relate to others
Guidance	Imparting of information and giving of advice by therapist or other group members
Catharsis	Release of feelings, leading to relief of past or present material; these feelings may have previously been difficult to discharge
Identification	Modelling behaviour of therapist, other group members
Family re-enactment	Group resembles a family and can give the individual an opportunity to deal with past family conflicts
Self-understanding	Development of insight about mechanisms underlying one's behaviour and its origin
Instillation of hope	Hopefulness about being able to 'improve', by seeing others improve, generates sense of optimism, that group can be helpful to that individual's situations
Existential	Accepting that one has to take responsibility for one's own life

Rosefsky do a detailed analysis of processes emerging in group psychotherapy with people who have a mental handicap, which compares favourably with that described by Crawley and is summarized in Table 7.4. The difference lies in the very structured leadership directives given by Szymanski and Rosefsky in order to deal with the situation.

It is important to note what makes the group setting particularly therapeutic. Yalom (1975) has identified factors, which have been summarized in Table 7.5.

These factors have as much impact in group psychotherapy with handicapped, as against non-handicapped, group members, and can also emerge, to a lesser extent, in activity-based groups, e.g. feeling of cohesiveness when playing sports; family re-enactment when preparing and eating a meal; instillation of hope, when seeing other people learn and perform a skill.

Running groups

Despite the wide variety of techniques from verbal to non-verbal, activity-based, etc, very similar 'rules' apply with regard to goal setting, aims, client selection, media used, boundaries set, use of group processes and leadership style.

The decision to run a group should arise from client need, from which the therapist can then formulate group aims, goals and how they might be best achieved. The choice of media to be used (e.g. verbal, activity-based, etc.) must relate to clients' skills, level of cognition, what will 'involve' them, etc. (e.g. Hodgetts, 1986; McGowen, 1986).

Many authors emphasize the need for therapists to be able to adopt an electic approach and use a variety of techniques in order to be able to 'meet' and communicate with the client at various levels (Gunzberg, 1974; Szymanski and Rosefsky, 1980; Clarke, 1984; Monfils and Menolascino, 1984).

Remarks made with regard to the selection of clients with a mental handicap into psychotherapy groups include: (1) capacity for group participation and 'social hunger'; (2) responsiveness to verbal and non-verbal cues given out by those around them; (3) a need to develop social skills; and (4) tendency to 'act out' rather than 'internalize conflicts (Clarke, 1984). Many of the criteria outlined with regard to client selection for individual therapy apply also (e.g. motivation, absence of acute psychosis, etc.).

Remarks about group size and composition are made too. the general consensus with regard to size is that 6 to 8 participants is most workable, but much larger than that, subgroups appear (Szymanski and Rosefsky, 1980; Clarke 1984). Attention needs to be paid to the number of therapists used – experience has shown that a group of 6 to 8 participants is more manageable with two therapists, who can take turns in leading, observing and modelling.

It can be useful to 'mix' group composition in terms of abilities and skills (Szymanski and Rosefsky; Clarke). For example, (a) more active and verbal participants may serve as models for the quiet and passive ones, and (b) in groups dealing with difficulties in heterosexual interaction, a mixed group of males and females can be useful in enabling discussion. Care needs to be taken, however, not to have too wide a range of abilities within the group – retarded adolescents can be particularly intolerant of lower functioning peers (Szymanski and Rosefsky).

As with individual therapy, boundaries need to be set early on in the group as to what is and is not acceptable behaviour and what the basic rules are (Clarke). This includes: (1) venue for group; (2) time and length of group; (3) number of sessions (if applicable); (4) limitations on behaviour, e.g. shouting, displays of physical aggression or destruction of the room are unacceptable; and (5) expectations in terms of input, e.g. setting up or putting away any equipment, tidying up afterwards. This must come in at the 'forming' phase, and applies to groups, both verbal and activity-based. It is worth noting the failure of experiments in group work with clients who had mental handicap that had a 'permissive approach' and were set up without any limits or rules (Vail, 1955).

Emphasis is placed by many authors on therapists utilizing group processes as a therapeutic tool (e.g. Gunzberg, 1974; Szymanski and Rosefsky, 1980; Cole, 1989). Peer pressure and feedback is useful in eliminating inappropriate and building up appropriate behaviours. It is an excellent venue to build up relationships between peers, which may be important in enabling other aspects of their lives to work more effectively, e.g. the group set up by McGowan (1986) prior to residents leaving an institution. Peer support and identification are very helpful in breaking the cycle of dependency – helplessness – depression – withdrawal; adolescents who have a mental handicap have been noted to be particularly responsive to learning that others have similar problems to theirs (Szymanski and Rosefsky).

Certain skills have been observed to help therapists in leading groups for people with mental handicaps (Szymanski and Rosefsky, 1980; Monfils and Menolascino, 1984; Clarke, 1984). As has been mentioned previously with regard to individual therapy, this includes practical knowledge about mental handicaps, flexibility in approach, and clear understanding for motivation to be involved in such work (Szymanski and Rosefsky). Monfils and Menolascino emphasize that: (a) the therapist's style and technique should be geared towards encouraging interaction and expression amongst group members; (b) allow for freedom and spontaneity, within limits, of communication in the group; (c) that communication must be clear, concrete and geared towards members level of comprehension; (d) that communication must establish and reinforce reality for each client; and (e) that the therapist should appear as a genuine, warm, accepting individual.

Clarke notes that therapists should be prepared to give a certain amount of self-disclosure and above all, maintain a sense of humour!

Specific applications of group work

It has been suggested that any activity involving a person with a mental handicap can be considered to have some psychotherapeutic benefit (Gunzberg) and that psychotherapy with this client group can be expected to include both verbal and non-verbal techniques (Gunzberg, 1974; Selan, 1976; Szymanski, 1980; Matson, 1984). On this basis, group work with people who have a mental handicap will be viewed from a very broad perspective, including those that are activity based, skills training orientated, use action methods and verbal techniques.

Developmental approach

Lederman (1984) examines group work in terms of developing skills in group interaction, which can be divided into five subskills:

1. The ability to participate in a parallel group, e.g. performing an activity in the presence of others, but not involving them;
2. Participation in a project group, e.g. sharing a short-term activity with others, with emphasis on task completion rather than social-emotional interaction and satisfaction;
3. Participation in an egocentric – co-operative group, e.g. where group members select, implement and complete relatively long-term tasks together, where the individual learns to have his/her needs met through meeting the needs of others;
4. Participation in a co-operative group, e.g. where a group of compatible individuals engage in mutual satisfaction of needs;
5. Participation in a mature group, e.g. where members assume a variety of membership and leadership roles, and attempt to both accomplish a task and to gratify the social-emotional needs of members (Mosey, 1970).

Lederman notes that group interaction skill is frequently deficient in people with a mental handicap, despite the amount of time that most clients spend in group situations, e.g. on a ward, in a day centre, in a class, in a sheltered workshop, etc. These skills are closely tied to the development of social skills; for this reason, Lederman then goes on to describe the groups that the OT can run to enable the individual to 'progress' through the various stages.

Parallel group The therapist must firstly ensure that a trusting

170

relationship has been established with the individual prior to introduction into the group setting. When the person is first introduced, the therapist should use an activity that is short term, simple and can be accomplished in the presence of others, e.g. individual craft project. The therapist, as the group leader, can shape and reinforce appropriate parallel group behaviour such as eye contact, casual conversation, etc.

Project group Short-term activities can be used by the therapist to develop 'project group skills'. Sharing, co-operation and mild competition can be part of this, which may be enhanced by simple team sports, games, group singing, meal preparation, etc. The therapist, as the leader of the group, encourages sharing, trial-and-error learning and group interaction.

Egocentric – Co-operative group In this setting, the therapist functions more as a resource person than direct leader and provides guidance only as needed. Appropriate tasks to use are long-term ones involving sharing, co-operation, problems solving and full participation of all members, e.g. decorating a large room or entire building for a special event, planning a party, organizing a fund raising event. Both the execution of the task and meeting of esteem and recognition needs is important to reinforce in this kind of group.

Co-operative group The therapist may initially function as a participant in this group, withdrawing to be called on as an advisor as needed. Activities noted to be most suitable for this kind of group are those that focus on the expression of feelings and social-emotional needs, e.g. projective techniques such as movement, dance, clay work, group mural, etc. The activity may be followed by discussion and feelings aroused by the activity.

Mature group Skills in this group may be acquired through any activity that allows or requires a variety of people to work together. The therapist acts as a peer, responding to the task and social emotional needs of the group as would any other group member. Mature groups that are community based include church groups, recreational organizations and civic volunteer groups.

This presentation of group work and group skills acquisition is of practical relevant to OTs working with people who have a mental handicap. Group type augmented by choice of activity can enhance social interaction skills. Parallel and project groups have the most relevance to people who are socially isolated, withdrawn, have a short concentration span and limited tolerance of other people. Higher social tolerance and communication skills are needed for the egocentric – co-operative group. Lederman notes that only a small proportion of the handicapped population have the sensitivity and insight to participate in co-operative and mature groups. While this might be the case in a practical sense, in normalization terms it is important for even the most disabled people to be seen to participate, if only by presence alone, in the mature group, particularly if it is community based, if only to remind the more able of his/her needs.

Furthermore, with regard to emotional sensitivity, whilst verbalizing feelings and making the connection between them and actions may be limited to the less disabled (mildly handicapped), none the less even the most profoundly handicapped person has feelings and emotions, which can be 'tapped' through appropriate means (e.g. Thomas and Howard, 1971).

Activity groups

For occupational therapists, the use of activities to achieve therapeutic gains with clients is central to one's professional identity, and activity. A constructive approach to the use of activities to achieve specific therapeutic outcomes in the group setting with people who have a mental handicap is described by Peck and Chia (1988). The choice of activity to be used is dependent on which skills the client needs to develop, to what media or format he/she best responds, and what the therapist decides should be the aim of the session. The therapist can 'check' that the selected activity is going to be of relevance to the set aims by analysing the activity terms of the development of physical, sensory and cognitive function, communication, socialization, self-reliance and work skills (Peck and Chia). Furthermore, these authors illustrate a set approach to group work that is activity based, by using 'group plans'. This requires the therapist to 'set-out' his/her approach in terms of: (a) activity type; (b) size of group and number of therapists needed; (c) teaching objectives; (d) equipment needed; (e) presentation of the activity to the group; (f) details about the activity; and (g) finishing off the activity.

Reference is also made to having sufficient time to prepare materials and staff prior to group sessions, presentation of the activity to participants (e.g. the finished product, verbal description, warm-up exercises), and having the activity take place in an environment that will enhance participation, in terms of room arrangement, space available, adequate lighting and room colouring (see also Chapter 4).

With regard to people with a mental handicap, the use of activities to achieve psychotherapeutic outcome in the group setting are described by McGowan (1986) and Page (1986). Drawings, pen and paper activities, magazines, music, clay and discussion are used to develop communication skills, enhance self-esteem, promote awareness of self and others and group cohesion amongst clients soon to move from an institution into a community home (McGowan). Puppetry is used to stimulate communication skills in the group setting (Page). The use of action methods is also described (i.e. the use of role play, rehearsal, performance and feedback) in relation to group work with people who have a mental handicap, particularly in relation to social skills training (Matson and Stephens, 1978; Turner, Hersen and Bellack, 1978; Stacey, Doleys and Malcolm, 1979; Matson and Senatore, 1981).

Groups are often the form in which living skills are taught. Having reviewed over 100 studies, Johnson et al. (1981) concluded that co-operation, as against individuation and competition, facilitated the learning of daily living tasks amongst people with mental handicaps. For example, Marholin et al. (1979) taught transport, shopping and restaurant purchasing skills of their clients in pairs, using a combination of modelling, cueing, rehearsal and social reinforcement techniques. The mutual support derived by the clients was particularly important in transport training, where towards the end, the trainer no longer accompanied the clients on the bus, but met them at a set destination. Matson (1981) in teaching shopping skills, used reinforcement from other group members to aid clients in achieving independence and to increase clients' involvement in the task.

Additionally, Tjosvold and Tjosvold (1983) note the particular value of peer interaction in developing social skills, such as co-ordination and co-operation in performing tasks and resolving conflicts in the small group home setting. Groups are also cost effective and time efficient. Even so, the therapist still has to have a plan/goal for each participant.

Psychotherapy and verbally based groups

Issues raised in psychotherapy groups for people with a mental handicap noted by Szymanski and Rosefsky include independence and plans for the future, discussion of one's own handicap, dealing

173

with inappropriate behaviour, making friends, sexuality, and expressing feelings. Hodgetts (1986) describes a (verbal) psychotherapy group where participants were encouraged to talk about their difficulties, getting on with others, and their hopes and aspirations. Although only a 'feasibility study', it is a good illustration of such a group, where particular attention is played to venue, and format and reactions of participants are noted. Interested readers should also consider Astrachan's (1955) description of a psychotherapy group with women who had a mental handicap.

Verbally-based groups where discussion and dialogue are the basis of skill development are also described in the literature.

In an 'exploratory study', a series of discussion topics relating to peer expectations and home life were presented to groups of adults with varying degrees of mental handicap, living in group homes in the community (Heller, 1978). The study demonstrated that peer group discussions and decision making (of day-to-day issues relating to the home) could be a beneficial learning experience.

An approach involving specific verbal interaction between therapist and individual members in a group, in order to counteract negative self-statements and develop self-confidence is described by Lindsay and Kasprowicz (1987). The presence of others in the group is used to give the individual feedback on his/her statements, in addition to any comments the therapist might make. It also gave participants practice at presenting a more positive image in front of others.

Groups set up to develop communication in and between individuals for people with varying verbal skills note both the skills taught (e.g. Makaton social signs) and emerging responses (Allen and Willet, 1986). The authors focus on the importance of assessment for the group (particularly the lower functioning ones), its aims and structured approach to sessions. Worth noting are the behaviours of participants in terms of the group life cycle, e.g. reluctance to make eye contact (forming); resistance in participating in activities (storming); willingly participating in dealing with a presented task, such as practising a Makaton sign (performing).

Other issues

Directiveness

The structuring of meetings and actively directing topics of conversation or tasks has been observed to be of particular importance for less able individuals (Szymanski and Rosefsky, 1980; Monfils and

Menolascino, 1984). Szymanski and Rosefsky note the occurrence of seemingly irrelevant comments being made in the middle of a discussion. For example, in the middle of a discussion about independence, one group member asked the leader, 'Have you been on an aeroplane?' The therapist must then be careful to strike a balance between directing the comment back to the conversation, through seeing its relevance to the individual. In the above example, the person concerned linked independence with air travel.

Connected with directiveness is the use of simple verbal communication, and expression of ideas in concrete, illustrative terms, and directive management of silences, which have been mentioned previously in relation to individual therapy.

Transference

Transference in groups differs from transference in individual therapy, in that transferences can be made with other group members in addition to (instead of only) the therapist (Slavson, 1950). The different transferences with other group members that commonly emerge noted by Slavson include: (a) sibling, both positive and negative transferences, such as jealousy and rivalry; (b) parental; and (c) identification transferences. The last is observed by Slavson to be particularly useful in group psychotherapy, and corresponds both with one of Yalom's therapeutic factors and Szymanski and Rosefsky's observations in working with mentally handicapped adolescents, who were very responsive to learning that others had similar problems. The presence of sibling and parental transferences links up with the group providing a setting in which the individual can express feelings/actions in relation to his own family (Yalom). The collaboration of 'siblings' (group members) against the 'parent' (therapist), can lead the therapist to find him/herself the target of hostility or aggression (Slavson). This links up with the storming phase (Crawley), and observations of handicapped adolescents making fun of the leader (Szymanski and Rosefsky).

It is important that therapists remember that transferences take place in activity groups also, as they can in many other situations, e.g. at work or at a social gathering. It is worth noting an observation of Slavson's that the family setting is most realistically produced when food is present. This is particularly relevant for OTs as meal preparation and consumption is a very commonly used activity. Group preparation and eating of a meal can be the ideal opportunity to gain some insight into how a person functions in his/her family

175

setting, but can also be used to engender a sense of 'family' and belonging.

Resistance, anxiety, countertransference and confidentiality

Although discussed with regard to individual therapy, these issues are mentioned at this point to emphasize their importance in verbal and activity-based groups. Even given limited communicative ability and severity of handicap of the client concerned, the therapist must take care that these factors are appropriately addressed.

EVALUATION OF THERAPY

In order to check that a therapeutic process being implemented to a client is of benefit and value to them, the therapist must perform some kind of evaluation. Generally speaking, this can be marked by 'pre-therapy' and 'post-therapy' scores, or by measuring performance outcome as against the aims and goals initially set.

Evaluation is noted to be part of the group planning process for activity groups (Peck and Chia, 1988), although it can be extended to be part of the psychotherapy group process (for therapists) too. Peck and Chia consider evaluation in terms of: (a) evaluation of each group session and (b) evaluation of client participation. Evaluation of group sessions requires the therapist to consider: (a) whether the group ran as planned and if not why not; (b) were the initial aims of session achieved; (c) could any emergent problems be dealt with more effectively and what changes could be made in the future. Client reaction is part of this process, and is examined by Peck and Chia in terms of participation, behaviour, attitude, interaction and engagement. Having aims and objectives for individuals in each session (as a part of an overall plan) can also be a useful way of evaluating individual performance and programme relevance.

Evaluation of therapeutic 'success' in individual and group psychotherapy has been noted to be very problematic in the non-handicapped population (Fielding, 1974; Gunzberg 1974; Fielding, 1975; Szymanski and Rosefsky, 1980; Matson, 1984) – these difficulties are magnified with regard to people with a mental handicap involved in psychotherapy (Gunzberg; Szymanski and Rosefsky).

There is a general lack of agreement amongst researchers as to what constitutes improvement, the reliability of the various measures devised, and ethical dilemmas associated with setting up control groups (Fielding). In an extensive examination of the literature, Gunzberg notes inadequacy of studies in terms of methodology and criteria used, and lack of follow-up studies. Despite the lack of scientific evidence to support conclusions with regard to psychotherapeutic work with people who have a mental handicap, he suggests that 'success' may well be due to the therapist taking an active interest in the client. Both Gunzberg and Matson note the importance of (the therapist) ensuring that any initiatives made in therapy are followed up by 'concrete achievements', implying that the therapist must have some definite 'administrative power' and weight in decisions concerning his/her client's future, e.g. ensuring on-going therapy, following up practical issues raised.

NEEDS OF THERAPISTS

Common difficulties encountered by commencing group therapists described by Dies (1980) and Spitz, Kass and Charles (1980) include: (a) management of the group (as against individual) therapeutic model (e.g. utilizing group processes, working with a co-therapist); (b) inability to handle 'problem' participants; and (c) leadership role. With regard to individual work, Buckley, Karasu and Charles (1979) have noted difficulties relating to: (a) therapist self-esteem and professional identity (e.g. wanting to be liked by client, over-use of intellectualization); (b) the therapeutic situation (e.g. inability to tolerate aggression or silence); and (c) therapist deficiencies (e.g. lack of interest or empathy).

These studies highlight the importance of good supervision and training with regard to the use of psychotherapeutic techniques, and this has also been referred to in Chapter 1 with regard to OTs working in the community. Dies notes supervision to be the most effective form of training for group leaders.

Gunzberg is very critical of the lack of supervision or experience of therapists who have embarked on psychotherapy with clients who have a mental handicap and considers this to be partly the cause of some of the more sceptical attitudes emerging in this field. Malan provides an excellent illustration of the supervision process with an inexperienced therapist working with a non-handicapped client (pp. 79–88). The occupational therapist seeking psychotherapy supervision need not necessarily seek out another OT. This is illustrated by McHugh and Knowles (1984) who received supervision from a psychiatrist.

SUMMARY

The use of psychotherapeutic approach in group and individual work with people who have a mental handicap can involve the use of a wide variety of techniques and approaches. These can be reliant on verbal and non-verbal techniques, action methods, art, and specific skills training programmes. This approach requires the therapist to look beyond the immediacy of comments and behaviours projected by clients, into their 'internal world', feelings and emotions. Such work has been done with people with a range of handicaps and disabilities, and despite the lack of scientific 'proof', it is both a useful and viable approach that interested OTs should use and implement, given supervision and training.

8

Integration into the community

Integration of people with mental handicaps into various facets of community life is the ultimate aim of community programmes and policies based on normalization principles. Integration refers to not only living in a home in the community, but also demands the use of public recreational facilities, such as swimming pools, or public bars, having work opportunities within the open employment setting, and making friends with neighbours, co-workers, etc. In terms of housing and use of public facilities, integration is quite easily achieved; it proves much more difficult with regard to social life and work, particularly given high rates of unemployment in the present economic climate.

In terms of helping clients to 'blend in' and integrate with others there are four main areas that the OT can become involved in:

1. Social and recreational opportunities
2. Employment
3. Education and
4. Advocacy

SOCIAL AND RECREATIONAL OPPORTUNITIES

Social opportunities

Barriers to social intercourse that particularly affect adults with a mental handicap include:

1. Poor personal hygiene (e.g. body odour, greasy hair, dirty fingernails) and unkempt appearance (e.g. crumpled clothes, fastenings undone, clashing colours);

2. Sensory deficits (e.g. deafness) and limited communication ability (e.g. few verbal sills, lack of sign system to use);
3. Poor social skills;
4. Inability to deal with conflict;
5. Inexperience in relating to members of the opposite sex, and limited sexual knowledge or understanding;
6. Difficulty in getting to places to meet people; and
7. Difficulty meeting people.

It could be said that these factors affect opportunities for integration for most people generally; they have been highlighted here in terms of people with a mental handicap as they are deficits which will make the individual appear more obviously different and hinder normalization integration. For this reason, they are key areas that the OT can target in a practical way through the institution of training programmes, in both individual and group settings (items 1, 3, 4, 5). (For information of training programmes, see Chapter 4.)

The issue of transport (6) is more complex, in the situation where the individual cannot use public transport independently and staff are unavailable to do escort duty. Given this and the difficulty in meeting people, there may be a great advantage in identifying a suitable befriender, to:

1. Accompany the person whilst he is travelling to a particular place;
2. To help ease him into a social situation; and
3. Be a friend to him.

This also gives the individual client contact with people from the community who are not staff or similarly have a mental handicap.

Using volunteers or befrienders is not always straight forward; people differ in expectations of the task, understanding of disability and have varying motivations for participating. Given this, it is important that volunteers/befrienders:

1. Are selected carefully (e.g. on the basis of an informal interview);
2. Receive some basic information about mental handicap – this should include definition, causes, normalization philosophy;
3. Receive clear guidelines on how often the client should be visited, kinds of activities that would be suitable, how to talk to the client; and

4. Receive regular supervision, either face to face or on the telephone.

It is advisable to also require a commitment from the volunteer for a minimum amount of time (e.g. six months).

Another model of social integration is through the setting up of a social or activity group for people with a mental handicap within an existing social club setting. This can have the advantage of providing clients with a secure base from which to explore other activities going on in the club in general and to mix with other attenders.

Recreational opportunities

Having surveyed the literature, Lyons (1986) notes a variety of factors that influence the ability of people with mild and moderate mental handicap in participating in recreational activities. Included are:

1. Lack of social and activity-based skills;
2. Limited experience and awareness of options;
3. Restricted opportunities by parents and caregivers;
4. Lack of local provisions;
5. Difficulties with transportation;
6. Prevailing community attitudes;
7. Lack of friends to do things with.

Barriers to social and recreational opportunities for people with mental handicap are ultimately linked and their solutions are similar. Both the use of befrienders on a one-to-one basis (e.g. Lyons) and a group setting (e.g. Shearer, 1986) are used as vehicles to enlarge the clients' recreational opportunities and experiences. Running groups in a community facility, such as a sports centre (e.g. Campbell, 1975), provides clients with peer contact and familiarization with a community facility, that in time may be used outside of group contact time. This also exposes the facility staff concerned to the client group, in a structured way, and may be a means to involve them with clients in time.

Particular areas that the OT involved in enlarging the recreational opportunities for clients should note:

1. Systematic identification of activities enjoyed by the client,

181

through trying out a variety of activities; the Daytime Activities Questionnaire (Appendix 2) might prove useful here. McKay (1976) emphasizes the importance of gathering information with regard to the client's past experience, amount of time available for recreational pursuits (in between work, day centre attendance and other commitments), general life goals, financial resources and transportation constraints;

2. Supervision and training of volunteers/befrienders used (see earlier discussion, but also refer to Gathercole, 1981a and Lyons, 1986); it can be useful to ask volunteers to keep a diary of activities done with the client, as a point of reference for such discussions;

3. Training of client in any relevant social skills;

4. Ensuring adequate preparation liaison exists with the manager of public facilities; this is particularly relevant when clients have an additional physical handicap and may need accessible toilet/ changing room facilities, or the use of special equipment in order to use the facility (e.g. a hoist to get into a swimming pool). It is important to check that adequate facilities are available at the time desired and that the facility staff clearly understand what the client's needs are;

5. Ensuring that caregivers are happy with the choice of befrienders/volunteer, and understand his/her function. This may require some time spent talking through any fears of letting the client go out, being more independent, etc.

EMPLOYMENT

Range of programmes

There appears to be two basic approaches to employment for adults with a mental handicap:

1. A sheltered workshop setting, where the individual can learn work skills and practices and then move on to an open employment setting with more support, and

2. Through direct placement in the work setting, where skills are taught 'on the job' (Shearer, 1986).

There is an abundance of literature describing various funding, staffing, training of workers, etc. There are centres described which offer training in work-associated skills, such as public transport training and social skills, and subsequent supported placement in a job (e.g. Blake's Wharf, described by Porterfield and Gathercole, 1985; University of Washington Employment Training Programme, described by Wertheimer, 1985).

Other schemes are described where a liaison officer actively solicits employers, looks for jobs that could be performed by an adult with a mental handicap, organizes any interviews, supports the person in the job, and in some cases, offers on the job training, until the individual has mastered the skills required (e.g. Transitional Employment Support, described by Wertheimer, 1985; the Pathway Employment Scheme, described by Porterfield and Gathercole, 1985; and Shearer, 1986; Geoffrey Rhodes Centre, described by Shearer, 1986).

In terms of direct work placement, other projects described include a craft work co-operative and bakery (Shearer), a sheltered work group, where a group of clients work in an open employment setting, such as a factory, as a group, and have their own trainer (King's Fund Working Group, 1984), working as cleaners in private enterprise (De Maars, 1975), and assembly work in the electronics and computer software fields (Wertheimer, 1985).

Work placement and projects for adults with severe and profound mental handicap are described extensively by Wertheimer. Work tasks noted include the assemblage of volume control mechanisms, circuit boards for home telephone systems (involving the use of machinery, such as a soldering iron), and defibrillators. The programmes described use the techniques of task analysis, chaining, positive reinforcement, cueing – visual, verbal and physical – as outlined by Bellamy, Horner and Inman (1979), and Wehman (1981) with regard to assembly and packing tasks. For further reading, see McLoughlin *et al.* (1987).

Important ingredients in a vocational service

In her review of five employment programmes for adults with a mental handicap, Werthiemer notes important features in programme design:

1. Well developed and clear aims and objectives, and a clear philosophical base;
2. Work-related aims and objectives (rather than general aims such as enhancing growth and independence), and a business-like

approach, as against a therapeutic or welfare-type model);
3. Great emphasis on meeting individual needs in terms of training, monitoring and placement;
4. Jobs that involved work highly valued by society (e.g. cardiac care systems);
5. Opportunities to meet and work with non-handicapped people;
6. Recognition given to the fact that support needed to be given both to the handicapped worker and the employer, and
7. Anti-discrimination legislation coupled with positive financial incentives for employers helping to foster employment opportunities.

From a wider perspective, essential components of any vocational service being offered to adults with a mental handicap, should additionally include:

1. Identification of individual employment preferences, skills, and support needed;
2. Individual support given to the person (e.g. emotional support, helping people to overcome low self-esteem, motivation, etc.);
3. Assistance with transport, e.g. public transport training, escort to/from work;
4. Links and on-going support and guidance to employers
5. Job identification, and placement, i.e. matching the individual to the job;
6. Job retention – support to employee/employer, practical assistance to the employee, job skill training on site, arranging co-workers to be 'models' for the new employee;
7. Flexibility in job design to cater for individual needs, e.g. height of table, lighting, need for jigs, cues, sequencing of the task (King's Fund Working Group, 1984).

Bellamy, Horner and Inman, (1979) note factors particularly important in keeping people with a severe mental handicap in a job. These have general relevance to more able clients as well, and include:

1. That individuals only be allowed to work independently in the production setting after she/he can perform the task reliably without errors;
2. That definitive verbal instructions are given to each worker regarding behavioural expectations and production contingencies at the beginning of each work period;

3. That workers should be allowed to devise alternative methods of assembly in production only if accuracy and production rates are maintained at acceptable levels;
4. Workers should be taught at least one acceptable way to obtain supervisor assistance;
5. Off-task and inappropriate behaviour should be ignored;
6. The quality of each product should be checked as soon as possible after completion to give the individual feedback and reinforcement;
7. Individual supervision contingencies should be designed for each worker.

Reasons for jobs breaking down

There is an extensive discussion in the literature as to the reasons for failed job placement of adults with a mental handicap, with varying degrees of disability. On the one hand it appears that poor social skills and maladaptive behaviour is the major reason for job termination (e.g. Schalock and Harper, 1978; Kochany and Keller, 1981; Wehman *et al.*, 1982), on the other it seems that poor productivity was the primary cause, with poor social awareness being a secondary concern (Martin *et al.*, 1986).

Other factors noted by Kochany and Keller which contribute to job termination include:

1. Inadequate attendance and excessive tardiness;
2. Parental reluctance and/or interference, e.g. failure to assist with regard to transportation and uniforms, frequent visits to the son or daughter at work, lack of understanding and co-operation with regard to social security benefits – that they will end if their son/daughter is on a full wage, etc.;
3. Supervisor vacillation in terms of job descriptions, attitudes, job performance evaluation and administrative support to handicapped workers;
4. Poor communication and transport skills, inadequate concept of time and functional academics; and
5. Lack of (referring) agency support, to the employee and employer.

Without extensive examination of research methodology used, it is difficult to decide which factors contribute the most to job termination, although all factors appear to undermine job placement, preparation, and on-going support and training of people with a mental handicap in open employment.

OT and employment

Assessment

Assessment of vocational skills is of four main types:

1. Psychological assessments, e.g. IQ measures, aptitude tests, interest surveys;
2. Assessment of motor skills;
3. A work sample approach; and
4. Adaptive behaviour and survival skills approach (Menchetti, Rusch and Owens, 1983).

The latter three are well within the skills of the OT to carry out and have the most relevance in terms of identifying individual skills and anticipated supports and training needed in order to survive in the workplace. (In some countries, only psychologists are permitted to administer psychological assessments; this is governed by a professional code of conduct and sometimes legislation.)

Fine motor skills Assessment of fine motor skills and upper limb mobility is essential if trying to assess an individual's physical capacity for manual work. Lower limb mobility is only essential if the work involves standing. There are various tasks cited by Menchetti, Rusch and Owens which test fine motor skills by requiring the individual to perform various assessable tasks (e.g. putting nut and washer on a screw) and use small hand tools. Examples of such assessments include the Purdue Pegboard (Tiffen, 1968) and the Bennet Hand Tool Dexterity test (Bennet, 1965).

In the absence of such sophisticated equipment to assess hand function as applied to manual work, the OT will have to rely on a basic 'home-made' kit, which should assess the individual on the following:

1. Cutting paper, cardboard, and vinyl with scissors/shears;
2. Using a guillotine to cut paper;
3. Putting a screw through a hole using a screwdriver (on a block of wood) and attaching a washer and nut; then the reverse of this process;

4. Picking up a pin, safety-pin, screw, and nut and placing them in a small box;
5. Holding a rod and pencil;
6. Testing grip strength, using a dynamometer;
7. Measuring range of movement at the wrist elbow and shoulder;
8. Measuring the distance the person can reach in front, behind and above (test by asking the person to pick up objects in these positions);
9. Picking up objects from the floor.

Such a test is not as thorough as the packages mentioned, but should give the OT a picture of the individual with regard to fine motor skills, grip, strength, and range of movement in the upper limb.

Work sample approach This approach allows the individual to participate in work by manipulating various tools, and displaying the worker characteristics the samples are designed to stimulate. The advantages of using such an approach to assess the workskills and training needs of adults with a mental handicap include:

1. The approximation of real-life work situations that isolate special skills within the reach of people who are severely disabled;
2. The assessment of worker characteristics (e.g. following directions, tool usage, attitudes associated with the work sample); and
3. The unbiased nature of the tasks, in that they are less likely to be influenced by factors such as insufficient motivation, anxieties language ability, and cultural influences (Sinick, 1962).

Examples of work sample programmes noted by Menchetti *et al.* (1983) includes the VALPAR Work Sample Series (1974, 1977, 1978), Vocational Information and Evaluation Work Samples (1976) and the Wide Range Employment Sample Test (Jastak and King, 1979). The MODAPTS assessment (Heyde, 1966) can be used as a work assessment test, in terms of hand function and management of loads in assembly work.

Adaptive behaviour scale and survival skill assessment This refers to assessment of social skills, personal care and community skills, such as money handling, use of public transport, use of telephone, etc.
    These areas are covered in many adaptive behaviour tests, such as the Adaptive Behaviour Scale (Nihira *et al.*, 1974), Progress

Assessment Chart (Gunzberg, 1976), the Copewell assessment (Whelan and Speake, 1979), and the Mid-Nebraska Mental Retardation Services Three Track System (Schalock, Ross and Ross, 1976; Schalock and Gadwood, 1980; Schalock, 1981), in which information is gathered either in an interview with the carer or observation over a period of time (usually days or weeks). Information needed may be gathered more quickly through thorough ADL assessment performed by the OT. The detailed assessments as listed above may be useful in terms of providing the OT with more detail. None the less, the information needed for an ADL assessment with regard to work skills should include information on the following:

1. Independence in toileting, eating and dressing;
2. Grooming, e.g. dressing neatly, able to brush hair;
3. Personal hygiene, e.g. using a deodorant, shaving, managing periods;
4. Communication skills, e.g. able to ask questions, respond to others, initiate conversation;
5. Social skills, e.g. getting on with others, ability to co-operate, accept directions/commands, problem solving etc.;
6. Use of public transport and telephone;
7. Money handling, including making small purchases, banking and budgeting;
8. Domestic skills, such as cooking and cleaning, which might be of relevance in the work place.

Skill training and work environment

The purpose of assessment is not only to reveal an individual's skills and capabilities, but to identify areas where she/he needs particular support and skills developed. This will indicate certain actions to be taken by the OT involved.

Skills training Assessment might reveal skill deficiencies in terms of work-associated skills, such as grooming, social skills, etc. Programmes to develop such skills have been outlined in Chapter 4 and are also dealt with by Wehman (1981).

Additional programmes of interest include:

1. The teaching of six job-related social skills – accepting a compliment, providing a compliment, accepting instruction and criticism, providing constructive criticism and explaining a

problem – through modelling, role play and practice (Whang, Fawcett and Matthews, 1984); and

2. The teaching of time management, using picture cues to depict lunch and break times (Sowers *et al.*, 1980).

The OT may also be involved in the job training, with regard to the best way to teach the task. The use of forward or backward chaining, visual, verbal and physical cues, and selection of suitable reinforcers are of particular importance with regard to teaching work tasks to severely disabled individuals (Bellamy, Horner and Inman, 1979; Wehman, 1981).

Work environment Another aspect of task acquisition is the environment in which the person is being taught. The OT must pay particular attention with regard to the height of the work table, type of seating and adequacy of lighting. Hand tools may need to be adapted if the individual has any fine motor deficits. Alternatively, there may be a need to design a special jig (e.g. to hold a component part in place) to enable independent completion of a task.

Other areas to consider

Pre-work programmes The OT may decide to become involved in pre-work programmes, with the aim of directing the individual towards thinking and looking at realistic vocational options, as well as developing skills relevant to the work place and general functioning in the community.

These programmes could take place at schools or day centres, in the case of clients who had missed out on such an opportunity in the school setting. Activities that could be included are: (a) visits to work places; (b) watching videos of people doing real jobs; (c) visits to job centres; (d) role playing interviews; (e) practice in filling in job applications; (f) learning about unions, health and safety at work; (g) learning how to relate to supervisors and co-workers; and (h) time keeping (King's Fund Working Group 1984). Such programmes are particularly important for severely disabled clients leaving school, if smooth transition into employment (be it sheltered or otherwise) is to be ensured (Wehman, Moon and McCarthy, 1986).

Wehman (1981) notes particularly the importance of teaching the following at the pre-employment stage:

1. Grooming skills;
2. Communication skills;
3. Functional social skills (e.g. eye contact, greeting responses); and
4. Leisure skills training (e.g. what to do during breaks).

Wehman also emphasizes the value of pre-placement job experiences, to test out skills and give the individual a 'taste' for work. This might be possible through some kind of paid scheme, although voluntary work could also be testing (e.g. helping out with a meals-on-wheels service, volunteer servicing/cleaning up at a community luncheon or programme for the elderly).

Voluntary work Voluntary work can be a viable alternative for some clients, given difficulty in obtaining paid employment and concerns about their standard of living. (In most countries, people who receive a disability or invalid pension are only able to earn a certain amount if they are not to jeopardize their income. Given uncertainties in the employment market, and fearing loss of a pension, which is often better than an unemployment benefit, the reluctance to give up a pension for paid employment has validity.) Voluntary work may also allow the person to work part-time, which might be more suitable to his/her temperament and needs.

People with mental handicaps have been involved in voluntary work, taking on the duties of carers, performing bathing, dressing and self-care activities for those more disabled than themselves, and presenting a range of activities to their charges (e.g. talking to them, making physical contact, providing leisure materials and music and taking people on wheelchair rides) (Realon *et al.*, 1986). Using such volunteers to stimulate others through conversation has also been noted (Dy *et al.*, 1981). The capacity of people with mental handicaps to perform these tasks can be confirmed still by older people who lived in institutions during World War II and were required to take on many of the caring tasks, due to staff shortages and/or conscription. If voluntary work is to be a realistic option, it must have many of the components of paid work, i.e. set hours, set tasks within the individual's capacity, on-site training, supervision and feedback.

Work options for people with multiple handicaps The area of work options for people with profound and severe mental handicap with additional physical disability is largely unexplored, although work options for people with either disability have been addressed (e.g.

Bellamy, Horner and Inman, 1979; Wehman 1981 and ILO, 1984; Schlesinger and Whelan, 1979, respectively).

There seems to be no reason why employment options should not be developed for this group of clients, providing that it fits in with other daily needs (e.g. physiotherapy, exercise, particular self-care needs, etc.). Any movement that can be elicited from the limbs, head or trunk could be used in switch control, given the selection of an appropriate switch (Oke, 1986).

Tasks that the OT may be involved in in creating employment opportunities for people with a mental handicap have been described above. With the exception of hand function assessment, work environment/task design and client positioning, these tasks are sometimes performed by other professional workers. For example aspects of assessment can be done also by a psychologist, as can be the training of pre-work skills, or task analysis as applied to the job. Additional tasks such as employer liaison and on-site teaching of tasks are often performed by a liaison officer, or specially appointed worker. This is not to say that the OT is excluded from these tasks; they may not be necessary for him/her to perform, if others are available, although attention and effort must be made in this direction in the absence of such supports.

EDUCATION

School programmes

The integration of children with a mental handicap into regular primary schools has become a more accepted practice, enforced by government legislation in some instances (e.g. in the UK – 1981 Education Act, Warnock Report, 1978 (Shearer, 1986); in the US State of Massachussets – Chapter 766 (Vaughn and Shearer, 1986); in Victoria, Australia – Intellectually Disabled Person's Act 1986) Integration has taken a variety of forms:

1. Direct integration in to the regular classroom setting, with the teacher supplied with special equipment/educational programmes;
2. As above, but with assistance of a special aide to work alongside the student;
3. A proportion of time spent outside the regular classroom, for extra tutoring in some subjects;
4. Joining the regular class for non-academic classes (e.g. sport and art) only;

191

5. Separate classroom and teachers for a group of disabled students within a regular school, with all students sharing the same facilities, e.g. play/lunch areas, some time for breaks, assembly, etc. (Shearer; Vaughn and Shearer; Gow, 1988).

Integration has also been applied at the secondary school level, although this is less often described in the literature. Shearer describes a secondary school project, where students with severe and moderate learning difficulties joined in with the other students for leisure, art and recreational programmes, but otherwise had their own programmes and special teachers.

Education for adults

As with school programmes, integration of adults into post-school educational facilities, such as college or adult education, varies with the level of ability and disability of the individual.

A programme that has been widely set up in London is a two-year post-school programme, usually set up in a college of advanced education (Shearer), where students use the college facilities, such as the cafeteria, sports area, library, etc. Within this setting, students learn and practice a variety of living skills, such as cooking, shopping and money handling, are involved in social skills development, sports and pre-employment programmes (see previous discussion), as a group. Occasionally, students integrate into mainstream classes, or receive teaching as a group from one of the mainstream teachers.

The main aim of the course is to develop student's skills further, and to provide them with an opportunity to come in contact with non-handicapped peers in a community setting. In some cases, the course enables students to move into employment. For others, moving to day centres is the only option, but at least the course has given them the chance to mature in a small group setting with peers their own age.

Wilcock and Lloyd (1984) describe a project where adults with a mental handicap were integrated into an adult education facility. Although they attended classes that were separate from the mainstream, they used the common facilities and were required to pay a student fee. Classes participated in included drama, yoga, literacy and numeracy, art, craft and music. More able students were able to use the classes as preparation for attendance at mainstream classes in other institutes. Tutors were able to support them when they moved, which sometimes involved transport training and orientation to the new facility.

A third type of adult education is the creation of modified vocational programmes suited to the learning capacity of people with a mental handicap (Andrews, 1983). He notes separate classes can give the student a chance to familiarize him/herself with the routine and expectations of the college and that such programmes set up through Tertiary and Further Education (TAFE) (College of Advanced Education) include woodwork, plant propagation, industrial machine sewing, basic oxywelding, farm machinery maintenance, tree grafting and welding. For further discussion on adult education, see Griffiths, Wyatt and Hersov (1985).

Separate versus integrated classes

From the projects described previously, a balance is needed between integration and separation in terms of classes.

Integration needs to be achieved firstly in terms of sharing of common facilities, and timing of classes and then within classes. Separate classes can give students a chance to familiarize themselves with the routine and expectations of the college and classes. This is very important preparation prior to integration. Integration at secondary school level of non-academic classes, such as sport or leisure, is a realistic way to begin. This could be translated into the adult education setting in terms of yoga, keep fit, dance, arts and crafts, etc. Depending on the student's skills, movement into more complex classes such as cookery, woodwork, or basic numeracy and literacy, should also be possible. In order to facilitate the move into integrated classes, it is likely that both the student and teacher will need support, in terms of what to expect, resolution of problems, etc. If entering a new facility, students will probably need direction in finding their way around, learning what facilities are available and guidelines of what is acceptable/unacceptable behaviour.

OT Role

The OT can be involved in a number of tasks which can facilitate integration in adult education. Where there is no integration, the OT should be involved in encouraging the relevant bodies to set such programmes in motion. It could be argued that ATCs and day centres could be less stretched if some attenders were organized to learn some skills through an adult education system, if given appropriate support.

OTs could also be involved in: (a) teaching classes in an adult education setting; and (b) helping individuals to move into the mainstream, by developing independence in public transport skills (or organizing a system of transport), social skills, and orientation to a new facility. Additionally, the OT may be called upon to assist with aids or devices if the student has difficulty in manipulating any tools (e.g. for craft, woodwork or cooking).

ADVOCACY

Basic principles

Advocacy is the means by which the rights of people with a mental handicap can be obtained and protected (Bruininks *et al.* 1980). People may be unaware of what their rights are, because of lack of information or limited comprehension. Advocacy, in its various forms, aims to advance and protect the rights of the individual, to obtain the necessary services and lifestyle which he/she requires and is entitled to as a part of the community.

Advocacy can be viewed as having a three-tiered approach (Herr, 1978). The first tier involves self-help, efforts of friends, relatives and professional helpers who may assist in obtaining basic services, e.g. social security payments. The second tier involves volunteer or part-time helpers who have some degree of training and can assist clients in obtaining their rights, e.g. a request for reconsideration of a social security benefit determination. Tier three involves full-time professional staff who can provide assistance and/or legal representation, e.g. a client's right to treatment. This is very much reflected in the existing types of advocacy services (see later discussion).

OT and advocacy

The occupational therapy profession is orientated towards enabling the individual to develop independence in daily living skills and exerting his/her influence over the immediate environment. Occupational therapy also enables the individual to maintain and consolidate the skills he/she has and a decent quality of life.

There is an emphasis on a person's skills, rather than deficits, in order to reinforce self-dignity and project a positive image of the person. The occupational therapy approach is very much orientated towards advocacy. By helping people to maintain and develop skills for themselves and develop a sense of control over their lives, self-advocacy is fostered. In this way the OT can make a valuable contribution to the advocacy movement. The OT can also participate in more formal advocacy programmes which will be described below.

Types of advocacy

There are three main approaches to advocacy – self-advocacy, citizen advocacy and state protection/advocacy systems (Bruininks et al., 1980).

Self-advocacy is the term used to describe both the principle and process of people with mental handicaps speaking for themselves (Griffiths, Wyatt and Hersov, 1985). It applies to people who are able to express themselves verbally, as well as those whose verbal skills may be non-existent, but who none the less communicate their views through non-verbal signals, such as body language, or a structured form of self-expression, such as dance or music. Many self-advocacy groups have sprung up since the 1970s, based in centres or hostels, or stemming from these sources. Various groups and how they are run are described by Williams and Schoultz (1982) Sang and O'Brien (1984) and Shearer (1986). Common elements include structured training in public speaking, listening to others, developing ideas, as well as support and guidance from a non-handicapped person, in developing these skills and setting up a viable organization. There are also various self-advocacy kits available, which may be helpful in starting up programmes, e.g. self-advocacy packs produced by Campaign for People with Mental Handicaps (1986) and Human Policy Press (1987).

Citizen advocacy refers to the use of a volunteer or nominated person to articulate the needs and desires for a person with a mental handicap, who is unable to speak for him/herself and/or where there is a risk of his/her needs not being met, unless there is some intervention made. This could include people living in hospitals or who are moving out into the community, those with little or poor speech that is difficult to understand or do not speak English (Carle, 1984). In order to be able to do his/her best for the individual, it is desirable for the advocate to be independent from a service provider or potential service providers. It s also important for the advocacy office or organization to be independent from service providers in administration, funding and location, and that the advocate and his/her organization have a clear understanding of each others roles (Carle).

Furthermore, Carle describes the advocate role as having two strands:

1. An instrumental role, in which the advocate solves practical or material problems, e.g. help with shopping, voting, representing the individual at individual plan meetings; and
2. An expressive role, in which the advocate is involved in meeting needs for communication, warmth and support, e.g. sharing significant activities or events, offering support in a crisis.

Advocates can be involved in either of these roles or a combination of both.

Setting up a citizen advocacy service should involve the following processes:

1. Publicity and recruitment of advocates through newspapers, radio, community noticeboards and subsequent information forum, where various aspects of advocacy could be discussed and presented by experienced advocates and service users;
2. Selection of advocates, based on criteria such as:
   (a) Positive attitude to rights issues;
   (b) An ability to network people into community activities; and
   (c) Valid reasons for involvement.
   Alternatively, potential advocates could pass through various screening stages, after an information forum, such as group interview plus one week training course, before ultimate selection;
3. Providing advocates with:
   (a) Training on the different roles and situations he/she will likely confront, as well as an overview of mental handicap, services available, normalization, integration, etc. (see also Sang and O'Brien for training programme content);
   (b) Support through training, on-going contact with other advocates and professional staff;
   (c) Evaluation, to ensure the relationship between advocate and client remains constructive and positive;

4. Matching advocates and clients on the basis of mutual agreement and after a trial period;
5. Evaluation of the whole project, covering recruitment, training and matching of advocates, structure and effectiveness of the organization, programme success from the client's perspective and support of staff/advocates and consumers, e.g. O'Brien and Wolfensberger, 1977; Dunn, Ross and Patterson 1984).

A third kind of advocacy involves formally-organized state protection and advocacy systems (Bruininks *et al.*, 1980). Protection and advocacy activities may be directed to individuals, organizations or classes, as a means to uphold the rights of people with mental handicaps. This is clearly illustrated by the recent government proclamation of the rights of people with mental handicaps in the State of Victoria (Australia), which clearly outlines and protects their rights (State of Victoria, 1986).

This kind of advocacy is very important in raising community and government consciousness, particularly in relation to making funds available in order to achieve more integrative programmes that will enable people with mental handicaps to exert their rights.

Problems in implementing advocacy

The introduction of advocacy, particularly self-advocacy, can have some profound implications for the community in general and those living and working with people with a mental handicap (Griffiths, Wyatt and Hersov, 1985). These authors note the changes enforced in terms of:

1. Professionals and parents needing to accept that people with mental handicaps need to be involved in far more meaningful consultation over decisions affecting their lives;
2. A change in attitude, with regard to the former, perhaps helped by training; and
3. Discussions/meetings proceeding at a slower pace in a simpler language that the person with a mental handicap can understand and contribute to.

The closed attitudes and narrow views of some professionals and parents are not necessarily changeable, and this can be a stumbling block in terms of advocacy and opening out alternatives to the client concerned. In many cases, the therapist must work alongside these

197

attitudes, particularly with regard to parents/carers, if contact with the client is to be maintained (see Chapter 9 for further discussion on families).

Another major stumbling block in terms of achieving self-advocacy is for people with mental handicaps being able to see themselves as adults, with positive attributes (e.g. capable of learning skills, paying attention, co-operating with others) as against a negative self image (e.g. lacking the skills to be involved) (Williams and Schoultz, 1982). The advisor to a self-advocacy group can help members to overcome this hurdle through accentuating the positive qualities and achievements of individuals, as well as encouraging a sense of mastery and control, and treating group members with dignity.

Citizen advocacy is only as good as its advocates are; therefore, careful selection and matching is imperative. The question of parents/relatives/carers is a difficult one, particularly in the case of an adult.

It is harder for relatives to retain an objective view of the client concerned, and in this sense they could be considered ideologically unacceptable as advocates. On the other hand, parents/carers can prove themselves very effective in obtaining the necessary and relevant services needed by the person they are caring for (Revans, 1975 a,b). In this situation, or in the case where an advocate has been rejected, the therapist does his/her best to make sure that the parent/carer and the client have access to relevant information and services, and in this sense, provides some advocacy service.

IS THERE A ROLE FOR DAY CENTRES?

The issue of maintaining separate day centres for people with a mental handicap can be extended to include separate sheltered employment and social clubs as well.

The existence of separate facilities at all would appear to be a contradiction in terms of normalization and community integration. However, closer examination reveals that separate clubs, workshops and day centres do provide a very real option for some clients, by providing opportunities for learning in a protected environment, and as a source of social contact. Kauffman (1984) has noted that social opportunities are generally limited for people with a mental handicap when they do not attend sheltered workshops or day centres. This reflects the difficulty clients can have in integrating into regular social networks in the community on their own, but also points to the social contact component which such facilities do have which should not be ignored completely.

Day centres can also provide a central organization for resources, which can be particularly relevant to people who are severely/ profoundly handicapped and require a variety of sensory and physical stimulation, and frequent input from various paramedical professionals. It could be argued that the home should be the centre of such organization, and indeed, this may be better if given good staff and community resources. However, it should not be ignored that time spent away may give carers, be they parents or care staff, the relief needed to enable them to concentrate on the task of caring for and developing independence skills, to whatever degree, of the client, at home. Home-based programmes also require staff to be available and have time to implement them; this may have budgetary implications in organizations where staffing is worked out on the basis that clients are out of the home during weekdays. Furthermore, day centres do provide a venue for clients to meet and socialize, the benefits of which would be neutralized in a home-based programme.

Separate facilities can provide a useful stepping stone for people to participate more in the community, as in the various programmes described earlier in this chapter. However, for this to be the case, activities must be based around the training of relevant skills needed in the community, and take people out of the day centre/social club building. In terms of sheltered workshops, community outlook can be fostered by:

1. Training in relevant work, and work associated skills (e.g. grooming, social skills);
2. Throughput from the workshop, with placement in open employment (with supervision and support) perhaps through a special scheme (see previous discussion), and;
3. The working including jobs which would develop the relevant skills needed for open-employment or be accessible to the client outside of the workshop setting (Kirby, 1986).

9

Working with families

There has been extensive research in recent years on the impact of a mentally handicapped family member on 'family life', with clear references to siblings and parents. Early studies have generally focused on the negative presence of a mentally handicapped member in the family and have been summarized in Table 9.1.

However, several authors point to poor methodology (e.g. heavy reliance on the survey method for parents and siblings, lack of control groups) and positive research outcomes which suggest the contrary view and highlight factors which do contribute more realistically to family problems (Crnic, Friedrich, and Greenberg, 1983; Ferrari, 1984; Carr, 1985; Peterson and Wikoff, 1987).

Siblings have been found not be devastated by the presence of a sibling with a mental handicap (Ferrari, 1984; Gath and Gumley, 1987), and are not at greater risk of psychological disturbance when they have a handicapped sibling, as compared with children who have healthy, 'normal' siblings. However, siblings of the same sex as the chronically ill child do have higher rates of maladjustment than do siblings of the opposite sex, although birth order has no impact (Ferrari). The ability of the family to cope is related to its own 'internal resources' (e.g. warmth, security) (Nihira, Meyers and Mink, 1980; Gath and Gumley, 1987), as well as access to resources, socio-economic status, other sources of stress and the severity of the handicap (Peterson and Wikoff, 1987). The adjustment of the mother to the situation is particularly important in determining the adjustment of her non-handicapped children (Ferrari). The mother has been identified as potentially at risk in terms of her health and marital adjustment (Peterson and Wikoff) although this should not be a foregone conclusion in every case. Not all families (with a handicapped family member) experiencing a high number of

Table 9.1 Some studies examining impact of a child with a mental handicap on family

Researcher(s)	Finding(s)
Farber (1959a, b); Friedrich and Friedrich (1981)	Negative impact on marital satisfaction and 'integration'
Farber (1960, 1968, 1970)	Reduction in social mobility
Bergreen (1971); Mattson (1972)	High stress, frqeuent emotional disturbances, and patterns of psychopathology in the family
Gath (1974)	Higher rate in emotional and behavioural problems of older sisters
Lavigne and Ryan (1979)	Siblings more likely to be withdrawn and irritable
McMichael (1971); Korn, Chess and Fernandez (1978); Freeman, Malkin and Hastings (1975)	Marital disharmony, physical and mental illness
Pless and Pinkerton (1975)	Aggressive and antisocial behaviour in siblings, that aims to get parental attention
Farber (1959a,b)	Younger siblings more vulnerable to disturbance

stressors experience adjustment problems; it should not be assumed that the birth of a handicapped child will produce a long-term negative outcome in the family (Peterson and Wikoff). Descriptive reports seeking out parents' views and feelings on having had a handicapped child further attest to this (e.g. Swain and Eagle, 1987a).

The usefulness of research is not merely in identifying features but applying it to work in the field. Ferrari suggests that therapists must endeavour to involve the whole family in any therapeutic approach, and will need to consider the needs of siblings and parents as well as the identified client. For example, the fostering of a social support network could be helpful to parents of chronically disabled children, and supportive discussion groups for siblings. This is also supported by Peterson and Wikoff. Crnic, Friedrich and Greenberg (1983), having surveyed the literature, suggest an adaptational model of family response, whereby the coping resources of the family are determined by the stressor(s) and the ecological context (e.g. friends, peers). This can be a useful aid to the therapist in understanding family responses to situations.

Close examination of the basic theories relating to family function can also prove revealing in helping the OT to determine action to be taken in the family context.

THEORIES ABOUT FAMILY FUNCTIONING

The two main approaches that appear in the literature with regard to the functioning of families are the systems thinking and life cycle models. Both have much to offer in enabling the therapist: (a) to understand family responses to situations, (b) to anticipate family needs at various stages, in order to (c) formulate an appropriate therapeutic response.

Systems thinking

Both Barker (1981) and Gorell Barnes (1985) refer to systems thinking in reviewing family dynamics. Systems theory, from which systems thinking stems, proposes an interacting relationship between a group of objects, be they organic or inorganic, in an open (i.e. interaction between the system and surrounding environment in terms of in-flow and out-flow) or closed (i.e. no interaction with the environment) system.

Families cannot be defined as a system with the same precision as an organism (Gorell Barnes) or the object, and for this reason the term systems thinking is referred to in relation to families. Systems thinking uses properties of systems theory to understand the workings of families (Barker; Gorell Barnes), some of which are mentioned below.

1. 'Every system has a boundary, the properties of which are important in understanding how the system works; boundaries are semi-permeable.' (Barker, p. 23.) For example, some families refuse help from specialist groups, therefore one needs to know how to negotiate that boundary. Optimistically, imparting information to the family is possible because the boundary has the property of being semi-permeable.

2. 'Family systems tend to reach a relatively, but not totally, steady state. Growth and evolution are possible, indeed usual. Change can occur or be effected in various ways.' (Barker, p. 23.) Family relationships and expectations change as children grow up, gain and assert independence skills, and leave to establish their own homes and families. Generally speaking, in families where there is a member who has a mental handicap, the situation often occurs that the person continues to live in the family home till parents die, and is restricted in asserting in any independence skills he/she might have gained (Flynn and Saleem, 1986). This is also a 'steady state' of a

sort, although movement may indeed be possible with the establishment of group homes, or when the parent dies. The indication for the therapist is to prepare the family and identify a suitable home, or resources needed to maintain the person with a mental handicap in the family home.

3. 'Communications and feedback mechanisms between the parts of the system are important in the functioning of the system.' (Barker, p. 23) That is, for the family to function effectively and allow for its members to grow and move, communication and feedback between the members is necessary. This assumes that family members can 'listen' and also 'hear' communications. Flynn and Saleem's study suggests that the listening and hearing of family members in relation to a member who has a mental handicap and wishes to assert his/her skills, is often lacking and unnecessarily restrictive to the person. Without wishing to apportion blame or guilt, the OT identifying such a situation could work with the family to consider that person's views, and help set up a way for him/her to utilize and express his skills in the family home.

4. 'Events such as behaviour of individuals in the family are better understood as examples of circular casuality rather than on the basis of linear casuality.' (Barker, p. 23.) This implies that behaviour of an individual in the family is better viewed in terms of a number of interactions and events which can continue to influence that person.

For example, Hussein's behaviour (Chapter 7) was related to a number of events, internal and external to the family – his father's illness, lack of security in daytime placement, difficulty in asserting himself in the family, etc. These issues were on-going and Hussein had to continually to deal with them. The task of the OT was not to 'fix' these situations for him, but to enable him to cope with them more effectively, by discussing his feelings and giving him some basic information, e.g. about death.

5. 'Family systems, like other systems, have the property of equifinality, that is the same endpoint may be reached from a number of starting points.' (Barker p. 23.) This means that the family may reach a solution to a problem by various means. It also implies that families do have ideas and solutions which the OT should utilize, and that the therapist can probably tackle an issue with a family in a number of ways.

6. 'Systems are made up of subsystems and themselves are parts of supra systems.' (Barker p. 23.) In the context of a family, this suggests that children, parents or the handicapped child/adult can all contribute as subsystems. Each relate to or are part of a suprasystem

as individuals, such as a school, day centre, or office, or as a group (e.g. part of the local neighbourhood). The OT needs to be aware of: (a) what subsystems are operating in a family in relation to a particular situation and how this can be broached to generate a positive outcome (e.g. rest of family versus handicapped member); and (b) where the family views the therapist coming from (e.g. a suprasystem of the handicapped member's, such as a day centre, or from the community at large) and to which family subsystem he/she is incorporated (e.g. parental, children, handicapped member, combination of all or some, etc). This is illustrated in a case study later in the chapter.

7. Homeostatic mechanisms operate in families (Gorell Barnes). This refers to the fact that families try to maintain a steady state during and after a disturbance. Its major importance to the OT is in considering what the likely effect of change in one member of the family will have on other members, and what action the therapist might need to take. For example, the impact of a person with a mental handicap leaving an institution and returning to the community can generate considerable parental/relative scepticism and anxiety (Halliday, 1987). By acknowledging the relatives' very real concerns, the OT can provide support and engage the relatives in constructive (as against obstructive) approaches to the various problems as they arise.

Systems thinking can be usefully employed in understanding how families work. The illustrations above relate this to the situation where a person with a mental handicap is involved and indicate how the OT can use this approach to decide upon appropriate therapeutic action.

Family life cycle

General reference to the family life cycle are made by Bentovim, Gorell Barnes and Cooklin (1982a,b). For viewing the challenges faced by families with a member with a mental handicap, Bicknell (1983) notes five main stages.

Breaking the news

This may occur early in pregnancy, given the availability of antenatal screening for some disorders, or at the time of birth when physical abnormalities may be seen. Alternatively, the 'suspicion' of the presence of physical or mental handicap may occur during childhood, as the child fails to reach expected milestones or odd behaviours appear. This may well occur before a formal medical diagnosis is made.

Irrespective of the circumstances when the family is informed that they have a child with a mental handicap, they are likely to mourn for the normal child, passing through stages as in any bereavement – from shock to panic and denial, guilt for one's part in producing the imperfection and, finally, acceptance. The various reactions of family members, to the diagnosis or handicap can be affected by: (a) the information received at the time of diagnosis, about prognosis, support services available, and the sensitivity with which it is presented; (b) sex of child; (c) social class; and (d) position of 'sibship' in the family.

Pre-school years

The care of a young child with a mental handicap is both qualitatively and quantitatively different from caring for a normal child. There may be difficulties with feeding, sleeping, establishing a routine, or the child may cry continuously or be unresponsive or be slow to reach developmental milestones. Parents may still need time to come to terms with their child's disability, and have a need for a support system to link in with, be it from a professional person, or non-professional support group. At this stage, parents/families begin the struggle with community attitudes and prejudices, to seeing a handicapped child on the street, and attempt to utilize community services such as play groups or crèche.

The needs of other children also require consideration, although this will be an on-going issue. Bicknell notes that at this time, parents will need to consider the risks of having other children.

School years

The child who attends a special school may be identified as different from his peers just because of that, or because of being collected in a special coach, or having to travel further than his siblings. (Even for the child integrated at a local school. Difficulties may be encountered with teasing from other pupils or reservation of teachers, although this need not necessarily be the case.) Evening activities may be difficult to find and family members restricted in their recreational pursuits. The handicapped family member continues to learn and achieve, but at a much slower pace which can be frustrating both for him/herself as well as the family. Support services, such as short-term care, parent and siblings support groups, or a sitting-in service, can be very useful to some families at this time.

School leaving and adolescence

At this stage, not only does the young adult with handicap have to face the struggle between childhood and adulthood, but he/she and the family must also contend with the change from children's to adult services, which will invariably differ with regard to personnel, organization and perhaps availability of resources.

With the onset of puberty, issues such as sexuality, social and recreational opportunities, asserting independence skills, dress and appearance, as well as propriety in public (e.g. shutting the lavatory door in a public toilet) can emerge. (This will affect those with severe or profound handicap to some extent also.) Daytime activities post-school may include a tertiary programme, day centre placement or employment opportunities (Chapter 8), each of which place different demands on the individual and raise a variety of concerns for parents.

Adulthood and death

The major issue here is the provision of support and care for the person with a mental handicap in the event of the parent/carer dying. Support in making decisions and setting up a practical alternative may be needed. Specific information may be needed by the client about death and what it entails. Bicknell particularly highlights the support needs of parents in the case where the death of the handicapped family member precedes them.

The life cycle outline can provide the OT with some ideas as to the context in which referral occurs. It is important for the therapist to appreciate some of the events both family and client have been through, and that problems have not necessarily emerged for the first time just because an OT referral has been made. Even in situations where the OT may feel the family are being unduly over-protective or restrictive, one must respect, to a large extent, the efforts that have been made thus far. Parental responsibility is likely to be on-going, unless a placement is sought, or the family is able to let go and allow the handicapped member to set up his/her own home, with support.

Within the context of the life cycle model, bereavement responses may occur with readjustments to be made at various stages of development (Hollins, 1985). Chronological age and developmental age may not coincide, which is particularly important in relation to puberty, and issues of adolescence – sexuality, transition from childhood to adulthood. While this may be related to the degree of disability, family attitudes and involvement are likely to infringe on the ability of the person to progress through stages in an adult way, as Flynn and Saleem's study would suggest.

Predictable problems for families

Berger (1983) outlines predictable problems that families with a handicapped member face; this fits in both with the systems thinking and life cycle models. He includes:

1. Making sense of the handicapping condition – what to expect, prognosis, obtaining accurate information;
2. Obtaining, locating, and gaining access to appropriate services – this is invariably an on-going issue through the life cycle;
3. How best to harness and use internal family resources to meet the needs of the handicapped person and other family members; often the family 'forms' around the handicapped person's needs being met, at the expense of ignoring other children's or parent's needs;
4. The stigma of having a handicapped person in the family, which might result in parents cutting off contact with their social network, becoming increasingly isolated and focused on the handicapped person; the family may be ashamed both of the handicapped person and themselves.

TASKS FOR THE OT

Having outlined two models in which the functioning of families with a handicapped person may be viewed, and mentioning some of the problems, the remainder of this chapter will deal with tasks that OTs (and other workers) will need to tackle in relation to the family of a person with a mental handicap. The importance of this is not to 'treat' the family, but to provide the client with an environment that permits him/her to exercise his/her skills and continue to develop. Any OT intervention will be likely to take place in the context of other support services being involved with the client and family. Bicknell suggests that throughout the stages of the life cycle, the family will need support in the following areas:

1. Practical and social support, via parent groups, voluntary bodies and statutory agencies;
2. Close relationships with other parents to share grief, milestones, etc.;
3. Professional help from general health and social services, although this may not be all that easily achieved;
4. Access to specialist services for education, some health and social services.

Hollins (1985) emphasizes, support services needed by carers, including social work input, counselling, practical help in the home, respite care, early intervention programmes, day care and leisure activities during school/day centre holidays and financial support and advice.

Aspects of working with the families of clients that the OT needs to particularly address are outlined below.

Presentation and response to the family

Recent reports on discussion groups held for parents of children and adults with a mental handicap indicate general frustration and antagonism experienced with professional workers (MacLauchlin *et al.* 1987; Swain and Eagle, 1987b). Specific examples cited include the medical profession failing to understand the impact on the family of having a handicapped member, of inadequate attention received in general hospitals, or of being unable to contact professionals at a time of need and being faced with an answerphone (MacLauchlin *et al.*). Swain and Eagle also mention that organizational barriers do not always help to foster the parent – professional relationship, aside from the fact that parents must respond to a number of professionals at any one time! Professional responses such as: (a) the use of jargon to obscure the truth, (b) judgemental attitudes about the parents; (c) denial of the extent of the disability; (d) omnipotence in decision making; (e) over-identification with the family; or, (f) collusion with the family's response do not necessarily give the family or client what they need either. (For further discussion on the dilemmas of parent/ professional relations, see Dyson (1987).)

Given these sobering illustrations, the importance of establishing a good working relationship with the family is essential. Indeed, it has been suggested that the response of professionals to the family can influence greatly their reaction and acceptance of a disabled family member (Bicknell, 1983; Hollins, 1985).

Techniques noted by authors that OTs should take note of include respect for parents, empathy and genuineness (Cunningham and Davis, 1985), and involving parents in formal assessments and sharing decision-making with the family (Hollins, 1985). From some of the criticisms noted earlier, other approaches whereby OTs could foster a positive relationship with parents/carers/families, include:

1. Avoiding jargon and using words or explanations that are more easily understood;
2. Avoiding the use of answerphones when possible and making sure that a person is available to take messages at least during regular hours. In the UK, emergency social work/crisis services are often available after hours through the local social services offices; whilst it could be argued that rarely the OT needs to provide emergency assistance; it may well be the case that the OT needs to act after hours if he/she is the key worker for a client/family, and also provide a system to enable contact after hours.
3. Regular contact with parents/families, by telephone, letter, or meetings and giving copies of reports or important letters.
4. Involving parents in some of your struggles and getting them to help you. For example, the OT and social worker were having difficulty securing a day centre placement for a client, and had responded by sending ADL and vocational assessment, and social work reports to the agencies concerned. The family offered to contact their GP to send a letter, as well as protest their local Member of Parliament. The parents felt in this way they were making a contribution and did not feel so helpless.
5. Being honest with families about what you think your client can realistically achieve, rather than avoiding the truth – the OT might need to be particularly careful in words chosen to explain certain facts and concepts.
6. Involving the family in any OT programmes set up – this might include selecting skills to develop that both the client and family agree need working on, and getting them to participate in the carrying out of programmes.
   Case example: The OT worked with Hussein (mentioned in Chapter 7) and his family to help him to use skills he had learnt

Table 9.2 Chart used for Hussein. (One chart per week.)

	Make bed	Make breakfast	Carry shopping (Saturday only)	Feed budgerigar
Mon.				
Tues.				
Wed.				
Thurs.				
Fri.				
Sat.				
Sun.				

at school and college at home. At a family meeting where his parents, brother Nihat and sister Pina were also present, several daily tasks were identified for Hussein to work on, and for various family members to keep him company: (a) making his bed (Nihat to to this also at the same time – they shared a bedroom); (b) making his own breakfast (Pina to do this at the same time also); (c) feeding the family budgerigar (Mrs M. to check Hussein had completed the task); and (d) carrying some of the shopping back from the market on Saturday mornings (Pina and Mr M. to do this also). The OT left a chart for Hussein and his father to mark off tasks completed, over a two-week period (Table 9.2).

After a fortnight the OT revisited and found that tasks (b) and (c) were carried out at the times required, although tasks (a) and (d) were a little more erratic and needed continued monitoring. Mr M. said he was making a new rule in the house that family members could only have breakfast if they made their beds. Follow-up some weeks later proved this new rule to be working very effectively.

7. Being sensitive to other issues with which the family might be struggling, e.g. financial problems, illness, unemployment, other family issues. It is important for the OT to assess that any

programmes or requests made of family members are not going to be an added burden. It is sometimes prudent to delay interventions until a time when the family can participate. the OT should also be aware of resources available to the family in order to direct them appropriately.

8. Regular supervision, to ensure 'on-task' work behaviour, that the client's needs are being met, and that one has not become enmeshed in family issues. Reference to supervision has been made in Chapters 1 and 7, and the importance of talking through work issues to another person who is not involved and able to offer objective advice is highlighted.

Sensitivity to cultural issues

In order to work effectively with clients and families who are ethnically different from one's own background, the OT needs to consider the following:

1. How well the family has adapted to their new environment, if they are new immigrants – this can affect the client greatly. For example, family members may be preoccupied with their own worries about having moved, making friends, seeking employment, understanding bureaucracies to the extent that they have reduced energy and emotional resources to give the handicapped family member, carry out programmes etc. Alternatively, the family may have integrated poorly in terms of making friends, understanding the customs of the host culture, and be very isolated. Eden (1987) cautions therapists not to use length of residency as a barometer for understanding various statutory authorities.

2. Language used by the client and family in the home, as well as comprehension of the host language – this may indicate the need for the therapist to work with an interpreter. Often children (who are learning the host language at school, outside the home) are used as interpreters, but this can inhibit both interviewer and respondent (Hume, 1984) and put undue responsibility on the child. Communication may also extend to: (a) understanding non-verbal gestures and cues, e.g. whether it is acceptable for a female therapist to shake hands with a male family member and which hand is appropriate to use; and (b) literacy skills, which may affect form filling in or charts being used (Hume).

3. Understanding of cultural rules and how they affect the way tasks

are tackled in a family sense, e.g. responsibility of all domestic tasks falls on the females or females are not allowed to leave the home unless escorted by a male relative. This can affect programme implementation, e.g. teaching male clients to cook and wash up may be seen as a cultural contradiction. It may also emerge that some family members may feel a conflict of values between home and outside it (Eden, 1987), as Hussein did (Chapter 7).

4. Learning naming systems. This is more complicated with people of Asian and Chinese origin (Eden), particularly the former, where family members lack a common surname. In such situations, Eden suggests that it can be useful to list family members in the following way:

Client's name: Nasima Begum
Father's name: Mohammed Ali
Mother's name: Afia Khatun
Family name: Khan
Religion: Muslim

With regard to Chinese names, the surname usually appears at the beginning e.g. Mun Wy Ming, with Mun, being the surname, and Wy Ming, the person's forename. Some women do not change their surname on marrying, although children take their father's name (Eden).

5. Understanding religions, customs and festivals (Hume). This can affect diet (e.g. observant Muslims and Jews who only eat meat that is slaughtered in a particular way), dress (e.g. modest clothing for observant Muslim females) and time spent away from work/day centres in order to participate in various festivals. For the OT, such factors can influence the teaching of cooking skills (e.g. taking into account the dietary needs), type of activities used (e.g. mixed swimming may be considered immodest) and when activities take place (e.g. to fit in with any festivals).

6. Understanding the cultural attitude towards handicap and illness; this can affect the OTs ability to implement any programme at all. For example, Borum (1987) describes the situation where a Indian mother took her 18-year-old autistic daughter to the local temple and was told by people there that her daughter's condition was 'her fate', to be lived through, and that perhaps it was a punishment for what she had done in a previous life. Similarly, there may be distrust for certain medical interventions, or total

opposition (e.g. Christian Scientists believe that disease can be cured without any medical input) or of anyone waiting to offer assistance in what is seen as a family issue. It may be that employment is viewed as the only acceptable activity for family members to participate in, and that hobbies/leisure interests do not count (Hume), which reinforces a negative image of the handicapped person.

Awareness of cultural patterns and expectations can enable the OT to structure interventions and home visits accordingly.

Communication

If the therapist has difficulty communicating to the client or his/her family, an interpreter may be needed. It is important not to let the interpreter get ahead of your questions, to make sure all communications are interpreted back and that the interpreter does not become too involved to the extent of giving advice or taking over the interview. The OT can usefully employ expressions and gestures familiar to the family to get various ideas across. It is important to use straight forward language and to eliminate expressions or phrases which may appear confusing or foreign.

Cultural acceptability of solutions/programmes

It is important to use solutions to problems that are culturally acceptable. This is illustrated by Eden (1987) in terms of eating, who points out that the obvious solution is not always the right answer. In most western countries people are taught to use the hand that is most convenient, irrespective of whether this means exchanging hands. In some cultures, transferring to their left hand for feeding is considered taboo. Dress is another area that can provide a challenge for the OT, for example the case of the client whose mother wanted him to look neat and stylish, but continued to buy him clothes with fastenings (such as buttons, zips and laces) which he could not do up. In her culture, clothes more easily managed by her son (such as tracksuits, T-shirts, trousers with elasticized waist) were considered sloppy and unacceptable. The challenge for the OT here was to find clothes acceptable to the mother so that the client could dress independently.

Any OT programmes and goals must fall within cultural bounds. Any independence skills developed should be the ones most likely to be acceptable, used and reinforced within the family's culture. For example, it is futile to develop skills in homemaking for males coming from a home where these skills are identified as strictly female. One may achieve more for the client in terms of his acceptability in the family by concentrating on tasks such as money handling, gardening, or public transport training. It may be more acceptable for male, as against female, clients to attend activities outside the home at night, such as attendance at youth clubs. This was the case with Hussein and his sister Pina, where Mr M. was very keen for Hussein to attend a youth club; only after much reassurance and a 'reconnaissance visit' by Nihat, deeming the club acceptable, that Pina was able to attend. Even though Pina was well orientated and could get to the club herself, an escort system had to be organized.

For programmes to have any chance of success, they must also be areas that the client and family feel motivated to tackle (see earlier discussion).

Using cultural and family rules

Awareness of cultural and family rules can enable the OT to structure interventions for maximum results. Fore example, in Hussein's situation, it was clear that Mr M. saw himself, and was seen by family members, as the head of the house, and as the person who set the rules. It was clear to the OT that for any intervention to work, Mr M. needed to be in full agreement, and that suggestions that came from him were likely to be the most successful. Programmes that might infringe on his position or authority were avoided, and the OT often sat next to Mr M. in family meetings to foster her 'alliance' with him.

Techniques used

Hume and Eden note the importance of using techniques when running programmes that fall within cultural bounds. Physical contact (e.g. in drama or role play) may be unacceptable, as are group work of any type, or sharing of feelings.

Key events in the life cycle to note

Reference has been previously made to events in the life cycle that are important to families in general (Bentovim *et al.*, 1982a,b) and specifically those where there is a handicapped family member (Rappoport, 1963; Black, 1982; Bicknell, 1983). At each stage there are specific issues that may emerge in the family context that the OT working with adults with a mental handicap will need to attend to.

Adolescence

Issues that emerge during this time noted by Bicknell to include transition from school to adult life, onset of puberty and physical maturation, need for social and recreational outlets, a form of occupation to be identified post-school, be it employment or day centre attendance, and planning for the handicapped person's future residential needs.

Given the range of issues here, the OT may need to respond in a variety of ways, either by setting up specific interventions, or getting other workers involved. This may include: (a) sex education, including developing an understanding about friendships, how to talk to people, showing someone you care about them, 'public' versus 'private' behaviour, managing periods etc; (b) assessing and identifying suitable recreational and social outlets and addressing any escort or transport needs of the client in order for him/her to attend; (c) assessing work skills via short-term job placement in holidays, or formal work assessment tool (Chapter 8); (d) assessing living skills; (e) using assessments to identify suitable post-school placement, be it open employment, sheltered employment, training in a specific skill, day centre placement etc; (f) following through any liaison work between children's and adult's services; (g) using living skills assessment as a basis for identifying future residential needs and contacting relevant agencies, e.g. social worker, residential services office, etc.; and (h) identifying any other service needs of the family, e.g. counselling, family therapy, short-term care, medical input, etc.

Moving out of home

Both the planning of a future residential situation and the actual move is a major event for both client and family, even if the client does not live at home. The issue of moving out of an institution into the community has been dealt with in Chapter 2, and various tasks for the OT identified. Action to be taken by the OT in relation to a client moving out of the family home is very much the same, although daytime occupation and leisure needs may already be set up. None the less it is a good time to do an overall review, to check that the client's needs in this area are being met. It is vital that the family is kept informed throughout this process, in order to gain their co-operation and support for the move.

Adulthood

Issues at this stage relate to the maintenance of vocational, recreational and social activities, particularly important in the case of an adult with a mental handicap living with an ageing, more dependent, less socially active parent (Bicknell). The need to plan for future residential options after the parent dies becomes more apparent, as well as understanding what death entails in a practical sense.

Tasks that the OT may need to address here include: (a) ensuring that present vocational, recreational and social activities meet the client's needs and expectations; this may necessitate reassessment of vocational, leisure and living skills and identification of alternative facilities; (b) assessing living skills in relation to future residential needs, contacting relevant agencies, and raising the issue with the client, parents/family; (c) opening a discussion with the client about death and what it means, the facts and practicalities; (d) encouraging the client to maintain living skills and develop others to enhance self-reliance and independence; client skills generally determine future residential options available; and (e) providing support to the client in the event of the parent dying, helping with the move to alternative accommodation if needed, working through the grieving process with the client (Chapter 7).

For further illustrations of the issues and tasks to be dealt with at this stage, see Bicknell's case report of 'John' and the description of Mary's move away from home in Chapter 6.

Indications for family therapy

The focus of this chapter has been on working with the families of clients in order to achieve co-operation and support for the therapist interventions with the client. It does not take a family therapist to work with a family in this way (Ballard, 1982). However, referral to a trained family therapist may be required to resolve issue(s) that disturb or 'block' the emotional development of family members.

Family therapy is very much defined by method, some of which are described by Hoffman (1981):

1. Structural approach – developed by Minuchin (1974), aims to redesign family organization, such that there are clear boundaries between parents and children and between each family member and another; the therapist is an active intruder, and changes the family 'field' by his/her presence.

2. Strategic approach – a term coined by Haley, which describes any therapy in which the clinician actively designs interventions to fit the problem; this approach is associated with the work of Watzlawick, Weakland and Fisch (1974). There is emphasis on identifying and following on the problem and symptom, and using the technique of 'reframing', whereby the therapist re-states a situation to the clients so that they can see it in a new way.

3. Problem solving approach – developed by Haley (1973) and bridging the strategic and structural approaches. Hypnotic techniques, such as 'providing a worse alternative' whereby a family is forced to choose between two alternatives, one of which is so horrific that they go along with it or think up their own solution, and paradoxical directives are used here.

4. Systemic approach – developed by the Milan school (Selvini Palazzoli et al., 1978), where therapists work in teams, for example male and female therapist in the room with the family and male and female therapist observing behind a one-way screen. Periodically, the observers may call either or both therapists out of the room to offer a suggestion or ask for more information; all get together towards the end of a session to come up with a recommendation which may be a ritual, task or prescription. Important theoretical features include positive consultation (i.e. rationale consistent with encouraging symptomatic behaviour, such as the family needing the 'sick' person), the systemic hypothesis (i.e. a hypothesis must be circular and relational), the uses of time, the referring contact (including other professionals and institution involved in the management of the identified patient), circular questioning (basic tenet is to ask questions that address a difference or define a relationship), and neutrality (which relates to therapists avoiding moral judgements or becoming enmeshed with family alliances).

Severe behaviour disturbances, inability to make relationships, distress signals 'sent' by family members are noted by Roberts (1982) as reasons for referral to a family therapist.

The OT working with a family can use a trained family therapist in the following ways:

1. For consultation in order to deal with a specific issue;
2. For on-going supervision in working with a family;
3. For management of a case, i.e. referring the family to the family therapist. (Roberts notes the importance of thorough preparation of the family being referred, by the referring agency.)

The situations where an OT should seek out the assistance of a family therapist include:

1. When the OT feels a particular solution should be workable but no progress is made with the family despite considerable effort;
2. When the OT finds the family dynamics confusing, despite having a good relationship with the family;
3. When the family dynamics severely interfere with OT programmes being instituted, yet the family still want OT input;
4. For the family labelled as 'difficult' by other workers, or when there is evidence of complex difficulties, such as rejection of workers, preoccupation with trivial incidents or denial of handicap;
5. When there is evidence of disturbance in other family members, which interferes with any OT input with the identified client.

Case examples of family therapy with adults who have a mental handicap are scarce. However, Black (1982) provides several case examples of family therapy with families that have a child with a mental handicap, which illustrate the practices and principles involved. For further general reading on family therapy, see Barker (1981) and Bentovim, Gorell Barnes and Cooklin (1982a,b).

SUMMARY

Successful implementation of OT programmes from the home require co-operation and support from the client's family. Some of the issues facing families with a handicapped member have been described and examined in terms of systems thinking and the family life cycle. In light of this information, various approaches that the OT should consider using when working with families, such as presentation, sensitivity to cultural issues and working with trained family therapist, have been described.

Appendix 1

Case studies

CASE STUDY A

The following case study serves to illustrate the processes involved in moving a client into community housing from a long-stay mental handicap hospital. This is viewed in three stages: assessment, active preparation and community phases.

Assessment

The assessment phase involved meetings with staff (including a charge nurse and librarian), and an ADL assessment (where a worker from the house the client was moving to also attended) which enabled the OT to identify the client's particular housing and support needs. A daytime activities questionnaire was administered to identify leisure and daytime needs.

The assessment phase clarified the tasks that the OT and client would need to complete in the active preparation phases. The case study goes on to describe OT involvement with this client in his first year out of hospital.

Assessment phase

1. Basic information

Name: 'Harry'

Address: Ward 4, Willow Hospital

D.O.B.: 6/4/1930

Basic information	Client	Charge nurse	Librarian
a. *General health*	Good, except for a weak right hand and leg which effects walking	Good; weakness in right hand and leg doesn't stop him from doing lots of things. Gets moody	Good
b. *Brief history*	Has been in this hospital for 30 years lived in other hospitals too since the age of 10	Admitted to present hospital many years ago and was abandoned by his family. Has had psychiatric difficulties in the past	Has been in this hospital a long time
c. *Important people* Close friends Family links	No contact with family since age 10; best friend is the librarian	No close friends on the ward. Gets on with the staff, especially the librarian. Thinks the other residents are 'inferior'	Pretty lonely person; likes working in the library
d. *How client spends his/her time*	Works in the library 3 afternoons a week; goes by bus into the local village once a week; likes watching TV, smoking and reading	Works in the library 3 afternoons a week; sometimes helps set tables on the ward. Likes talking to staff, watching TV and going shopping. Often reads	Helps out in the library 3 times a week - puts books back on shelves helps with cataloguing. A very good talker, likes to be helpful and enjoys reading

e. *Additional information from case records*

Has been in institutions since age 10; age 10-20 years lived in mental handicap institution 'X'; age 20-25 transferred to 'Y' psychiatric hospital because of violent behaviour; was diagnosed as having 'paranoid personality disorder'. Then, aged 15 transferred to present hospital. No longer physically abusive to others but can be very aggressive verbally. No family contact. Can be very pleasant person, when in good mood. Has lots of skills and potential for community living.

2. ADL assessment

ADL assessment	Assessor's observations	Charge Nurse	Librarian
a. *Mobility* Walking Stairs Transfers sitting to standing and vice versa in/out bed in/off toilet in/out bath Any mobility aids e.g. wheelchair, frame	Independent in all areas; needs bannister to hold onto when going up- or downstairs	Independent in all these areas	Walks with no difficulty; don't know about other areas
b. *Feet* Type of shoe Any oedema in legs	Flat, can't do up laces; no bows or slip-ons required	Has trouble doing up laces, staff to do this for him	Often laces aren't done up
c. *Bathing* Washing, front, back, hair, feet Any aids used, e.g. bath mat, rail	Independent Needs to grab rail to hold on to	Completely independent	Don't know
d. *Toilet* Knows when to go Continence Any aids used e.g. rail	Independent	Completely independent	No problems
e. *Dressing* Top half of body Bottom half of body Shoes and socks Any aids used	Independent; main problem is doing laces on shoes and buttons on his left cuff on shirt	Can't do up left cuff on shirt and shoe laces otherwise, no problems	No problems apart from shoe laces

2. ADL assessment contd.

ADL assessment	Assessor's observations	Charge Nurse	Librarian
f. Eating Feeding self Holding cup/drink Any aids used	Has difficulty cutting food with standard knife; could use splayde and non-slip mat	Food is cut up for him; otherwise, has no difficulties	Don't know
g. Personal hygiene Cleaning teeth Brushing hair Shave Manage periods	Not assessed but says he does these without difficulty Not applicable	Can do all of these but not always very motivated	Don't know
h. Other skills Money handling Writing letters Telling time Using telephone Public transport Other	Recognizes coins; can do simple calculations Writes slowly can sign name Can tell time Can speak on telephone but can't dial Says he uses a local bus once a week to go to village	Often goes to the hospital shop Can sign name Can tell time Can answer the telephone Uses local bus service	Writes well, can read - likes spy novels Use local bus service
i. Communication skills Initiates conversation No speech Responds to questions asked Interaction with others Words used Any sign systems, e.g. Makaton, Rebus	Very chatty, asks questions freely, will respond to questions. Is very articulate	Likes talking, very articulate person	Will initiate conversation; has a good sense of humour; speaks well on the telephone (often answers it when in the library)

3. Domestic and Living skills assessment

The assessment revolved around making beans on toast and tea. As a result of the session, the OT identified that;

1. Harry could not open a tin using a conventional opener; he could manage, with instruction, to use an electric can opener;
2. He could not butter bread if it was flat on a plate; he could manage this task, though, with a small board with a raised edge on two sides, to push the bread against;
3. He could chop 'soft' vegetables such as tomatoes on an ordinary chopping board, but found it easier if a non-slip mat was placed underneath. A spike board was needed to chop 'harder' vegetables such as potatoes or carrots, and a broad-handled vegetable peeler required to peel them;
4. Harry could wash dishes independently, although he complained of feeling tired; a perch stool was found to be useful here;
5. Harry made tea without any difficulty at all;
6. He had no difficulty opening a door lever handle, the refrigerator or the oven or turning on/off light switches, the gas cooker and the water taps;
7. He could make a bed.

Given the results of the ADL and domestic assessment it was clear that the following would be required:

1. Kitchen and eating aids – including a spike board, broad-handled peeler, non-slip mat, a splayde, an electric tin opener, a perch stool and a bread-and-butter board;
2. Dressing aids – 'no-bows' could be used for shoes with laces (in future Harry should be encouraged to buy 'slip-on' shoes); the buttons on Harry's left shirt sleeves could be sewn on with fine hat elastic and the button kept done up permanently (the elastic would allow for the cuff to expand when Harry puts his hand through it);
3. Bathing aids – a rail would be needed next to the bath, for Harry to steady himself on when getting out of the bath.
4. Seating – any lounge chair purchased should have a supportive back, solid armrests and no lower than 45 cm from the ground.

4. *Housing and support needs*

From the information gathered from the previous assessment, the OT was able to note Harry's housing needs (see housing checklist). It was apparent that ground floor accommodation would be preferable but not essential. The only feature of note was the requirement for a grab rail beside the bath. Harry particularly wanted to have his own room that he could furnish as he wished. He had no special friends he wished to live with, but said he would like to be with people his own age. It was envisaged that he would need a lot of support initially to get into a domestic routine and to organize activities to do during the day. But it was anticipated that support could be reduced in time.

Client's name: 'Harry'   OT: Debbie Isaac   Date:

Household features	Comments
1. Household type (ground floor, two storey, flat, house)	Ground floor preferred; if stairs no more than one storey preferred
2. Entrances. (ramp, threshold flush)	Standard
3. Width – door ways	Standard
– passage ways (900 mm min. for wheelchair users)	Standard
4. Height – light switches	Standard
door handles	Standard
socket outlets	Standard
window openers	Standard
telephone	Standard
5. Type – light switch	Standard
door handle	Standard
window openers	Standard
telephone	Standard
floor coverings	Standard
doors	Standard
door closers	Standard
taps	Standard
6. Placement of fire blanket, fire extinguisher, height fire alarm	Within client's reach
7. Bathroom – size	
– bath or shower, siting of bath or shower	Bath preferred, sited along side a wall, to enable a rail to be attached
– rails/other aids	
– wash basin	
– cantilevered or other	Standard
– siting	
– flooring	
– type	Non-slip

Household features	Comments
8. Toilet area - size - rails/other aids - siting of toilet bowl - wash basin - cantilevered or other - siting	Standard Standard Standard Standard
9. Kitchen - height of sink, work areas and cupboards - special selection required for stove, refrigerator, washing machine	Standard Standard Simple controls: should be purchased with client
10. Bedroom - easy access to bathroom/toilet - size - call button - special features (e.g. strong joints)	No special needs noted

Further comments: Site visit with client required

5. Harry's occupational and leisure needs

One of the support workers helped Harry to fill in the questionnaire. The following activities were identified as those Harry wanted to pursue once he moved:

- going for walks
- using buses to explore the surrounding suburbs
- going to pubs and cafés
- watching TV
- borrowing books from the library
- getting a job, perhaps helping out in a library
- meeting people.

Active preparation phase

1. Housing

A two-bedroom flat on the ground floor of a three-storey house was identified as a possible place for Harry to live (Fig. 5.3). It was owned by a housing association and had been recently refurbished. The other flat (on the top two floors) was also to be let to two people with mental handicaps.

225

Another man from the hospital, Joey, was identified as someone whom Harry could live with. The support workers began to get the two men together on a regular basis and they seemed to get on well.

A site visit was made with the two men and neither had any difficulties getting around the flat or opening doors and cupboards. As both men were unsteady getting in/out of the bath, it was clear that a grab rail had to be placed on the wall alongside the bath. The OT put in a request to the housing association for this to be done. A cooker and washing machine had to be purchased so the relevant dimensions were taken.

2. ADL/Domestic/Living skills

Various appliances and equipment were ordered from the local social services department. This included a spike board, broad-handled peeler, non-slip mat, a spade, and electric tin opener, a perch stool and bread-and-butter board.

The support workers went shopping with Harry (and Joey) to buy the cooker, kitchen equipment and bedding. Sessions in the training department at the hospital were organized three times a week for the staff and two men to meet and 'do' things together, for example making lunch or visiting the nearby village by bus, to go shopping or have lunch in a cafe.

3. Leisure and occupational tasks

The support workers brought Harry up to his new neighbourhood once a week, with the help of the volunteer driver. Local shops and cafe were investigated, and a visit was made to the local library. The OT decided not to actively pursue job opportunities for Harry till after he moved.

4. Final stage

The bath rail was fitted and deemed suitable by the OT. On a visit to the house, Harry tried it himself and found the rail very helpful. The various appliances were purchased and delivered. The OT arranged for the social services department to deliver the ordered equipment on the day the two men moved in. The cooker and the telephone were installed at this time. Together with the hospital staff, the support workers and Harry also finalized the necessary paperwork required in order to receive his social security benefit at his new address.

Community Phase

Unfortunately, the flat was not completely organized and fitted out by the time Harry moved. This made the first few months that much more stressful.

Early tasks

Harry had not yet found a suitable lounge chair that was within his budget; fortunately his support worker located a very good second-hand furniture shop nearby that had a range of chairs, one of which suited Harry's needs. (In time Harry made several purchases from the shop and became 'friends' with the shopkeeper.) The washing machine had not been purchased; the OT went shopping with Harry and Joey to choose an appliance, and selected a front-loading machine with push-button controls. Unfortunately, until the machine arrived, the care staff and clients spent a good deal of time at the laundromat.

Harry continued to have difficulties with his finances; he did not automatically receive the correct benefits that he was entitled to, and this meant he had very little spending money. As it transpired, he was very nervous about handling money, and consistently required help from staff for banking and budgeting, although he was able to make small purchases from shops. Care staff accompanied him and Joey when they did their weekly shopping at the supermarket.

Domestic activities

Harry made his own breakfast each day, but was less motivated to prepare midday and evening meals. Care staff helped Harry in this respect. He was even less interested in cleaning up the kitchen or the bathroom, which brought him into conflict with Joey. The OT and support worker decided to set out a time table to be agreed by Harry as to dates and times he would do his chores. Unfortunately he needed constant reminders to fulfil this agreement.

Day-time needs

Having been very busy in the first couple of months setting up the house, and getting to know the neighbourhood, Harry became increasingly unmotivated to do anything. He slept in till midday and complained of not having anything to do. He expressed an interest

227

in doing some classes, and his support worker helped to enrol him in local history and old time dancing classes. Harry was very enthusiastic at first but after a while lost interest.

After discussion with the OT, the support worker contacted a volunteer services co-ordinator about possible volunteer jobs for Harry. Harry went for an interview and was very pleased about having the opportunity to do some work. He got a part-time job, three days a week, doing simple gardening at a hostel for physically handicapped children. He went to and from the hostel by bus and seemed to be quite happy for a few weeks. Then he began sleeping in again, and losing interest.

On contact with the hostel, it transpired that he was hardly working, and that they had not given him much supervision. Harry had been spending a lot of time drinking tea in the hostel kitchen. The job was terminated, but Harry was still keen to spend his time constructively. (He had, in the meantime, joined a local club, was going to the library once a week, and visiting his friend at the second-hand shop regularly.)

The OT then contacted several people who helped to organize paid and voluntary work for people with mental handicaps. Harry came to a meeting where his situation was discussed. He was keen to get some library work, and it appeared that there was some voluntary work needed at the local Salvation Army library. It was felt that the librarian would be sufficiently sympathetic to Harry, and give him time to talk and the supervision he required to do the task. He commenced at the library once a week, and at the time of writing, was quite content there.

Challenges for the OT

Harry was continuing to ask staff to do up his shoe laces and left shirt cuff. The OT and Harry agreed that the problem could be resolved by using no-bows on the shoes and sewing the cuff button with hat elastic. (The cuff could remain done up and the elastic would allow for 'give' when Harry put his hand through.) Harry was shown how to use the no-bows, and was able to tie them competently. One of the support workers agreed to sew the buttons for Harry.

All the support staff were informed of these new 'devices' being used by Harry, but he persistently requested help from the support staff. The OT reminded Harry how the devices worked and he again reiterated that he though it would enable him to be more independent. A week later he was still asking for help. The OT sat down with Harry and the house leader and they all agreed now that Harry had no problems with the cuff or shoes provided he followed the instructions. Both the OT and Harry signed a simple contract to confirm this. The support staff agreed not to help Harry with these tasks and reminded him that he could do them by himself.

Harry had difficulty using the public telephone in the hall; he could not dial and hold the telephone receiver at the same time as he only had the use of his left hand. He could not tuck the receiver under his chin, and the receiver rests commercially available were unsuitable. The OT ordered a telephone amplifier, that could be placed on a table next to the telephone. This would enable Harry to put the receiver on the amplifier then dial with his left hand.

The front door was also proving to be difficult. The lock was too high for Harry to reach comfortably, and as it had no handle, it had to be pushed. The OT and Harry went to a hardware shop and selected a suitable handle to replace the existing one.

Attention-seeking Behaviour

Harry's attention-seeking behaviour was very difficult to manage. His relationship with Joey had deteriorated, and they were no longer sharing meals together. Harry was verbally abusive to him, and made racist remarks to the black and Jewish personnel working in the house.

The support staff, OT and psychologist met to devise a strategy to deal with Harry's behaviour. It was agreed that when he was abusive to staff, he would be given 15 minutes to cool down, then staff would approach him again, and repeat this procedure until he had calmed down. All those in contact with Harry agreed to follow this procedure.

To deflect his attention-seeking behaviour, it was suggested that one of the staff spend half an hour with him every evening, just to talk about his interests, etc. It was felt also that he would be less attention seeking if living in a more stimulating environment, with a number of people (four or five). The OT agreed to bring this to the attention of the team administrator involved in housing development. But as there were still people to move from the hospital, it was unlikely there could be any suitable accommodation in the future.

The group continued to meet, to renew the strategies and also to give mutual support. By this stage, Harry had been living in the community for one year.

CASE STUDY B

This is included to demonstrate the use of assessment in identifying a profoundly handicapped young man's care, housing, social, leisure and occupational needs.

David was a 24-year-old man who had both profound mental handicap, cerebral palsy, and petit mal epilepsy. Assessment by the OT revealed the following with regard to ADL:

1. *Mobility* – he was unable to walk with assistance, dependent on staff for all transfers, had poor postural control and his body flopped forward, if unsupported. He sat (and was wheeled around in) a moulded seat on top of a wheelchair and had insufficient arm control (and probably cognition skills) to wheel himself around. David was happiest lying on the floor (in prone) with a wedge placed underneath the top half of his body. (He spent some time like this each day, as well as in a standing frame when he attended physiotherapy.) He had attended hydrotherapy sessions in the past and enjoyed these immensely, but this had been discontinued due to staff shortages.
2. *Bathing* – dependent on staff; bathed in a bath insert placed on top of a regular bath which is light to lift.
3. *Dressing* – completely dependent on assistance here; is dressed on top of the bed.
4. *Toileting* – is doubly incontinent and nappies are used.
5. *Eating and drinking* – is fed mushy foods by staff; reaches out to food as it was being placed in his mouth. Possibly this action could be encouraged with a built up handle on his spoon, as well as cup with handles on both sides for drinking.
6. *Communication skills* – has no sign system; smiles when people talk to him; difficult to know how much he comprehends.

Given this information, the OT was able to identify this young man's housing and support needs. It was clear he needed support in all aspects of daily living, opportunities for stimulation and activity, and therefore would need to have 24-hour staff support. He needed to live in ground floor accommodation that was wheelchair accessible throughout, and fairly spacious, as his moulded seat was wide. Also, it was anticipated that he might spend some time in his standing frame, particularly so that he could look on in activities, such as cooking, where he was unable to participate. It was difficult to anticipate whether a shower or a bath would be more useful, without a site visit.

Figure A.1 (a), (b) David's house. (With thanks to Habinteg Housing Association.)

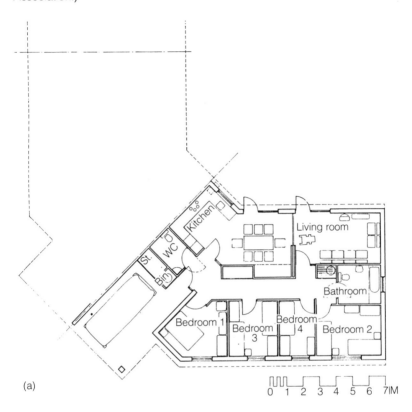

(a)

0 1 2 3 4 5 6 7|M

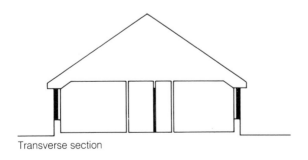

Transverse section

(b)

Figure A.2 Shower frame to be placed over the bath for David's use. (Not drawn to scale.)

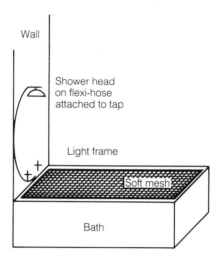

Wall

Shower head
on flexi-hose
attached to tap

Light frame

Soft mesh

Bath

A property became available that was both spacious and wheelchair accessible throughout (Figure A.1). A site visit revealed that: (a) the doorways to David's bedroom and to the lounge (from the hallway) needed widening, and (b) a shower frame was needed over the bath (Figure A.2), so that David could lie on this and be showered with a hand hose. (The bath was too short for a bath insert.) The bath was low and the OT was concerned that care staff should keep any lifting of David to a minimum. For this reason the shower frame was suggested, so that David could lie on this and be showered with a hand-held hose.

Appendix 2

Daytime activities questionnaire

AIMS

The following questionnaire was used by the North Southwark CMHT to establish the need for various daytime opportunities and facilities for clients moving out of a long-stay mental handicap institution into the community.

The aim of the survey was to establish:

1. The number of required day centre and adult education places needed;
2. The number of people wanting to work;
3. The need for volunteers, befrienders;
4. The leisure interests of clients.

This information was vital in order to 'bid' for money to establish resources to fulfil these demands, and to negotiate with the local authority for day centre places.

If anything, it yielded an *underestimation* of services, given that most of the clients interviewed only had vague notions about some of the activities, due to 'underexposure' in the institutional setting. With more time spent with the client after the move, carers would have a better idea of the client's interests.

ADMINISTERING THE QUESTIONNAIRE

The questionnaire should be administered to the clients by as few interviewers as possible, to ensure consistency in the posing of questions. Given time constraints, the questionnaire could also be administered by the client's keyworker/advocate. This may not yield a scientifically valid result, but may be an option worth considering if the information has to be gathered in a hurry.

The client him/herself should be interviewed but, for those less verbally skilled, with a person who knows him/her well, such as a key worker or advocate, present. This is particularly important where a communication system, such as Makaton or a communication board is used. Sometimes the keyworker/advocate will have to answer all the questions on behalf of the client if he/she can't answer. The disadvantage of having to use another person to help the client answer is that questions might be altered or rephrased. If the interviewer is concerned that he/she is receiving unreliable responses from the client on the Yes/No answers to questions 3-6, he/she should question the client, 'How often do you do (x)?'

e.g. Interviewer: Do you go swimming now?
     Client: Yes.
     Interviewer: How often do you go swimming?
     Client: I went once last year.

APPLICATIONS OF QUESTIONNAIRE

The questionnaire is by no means an empirical measure; what is presented here is a *modified* form of the original questionnaire. It is a suggested format for collecting information on daytime needs of clients moving out of long-stay mental handicap hospitals. It could also be used with clients, with mental handicaps, who are already living in the community, but the following modifications should be made:

1. With regard to questions 3-6, if the respondent answers 'yes', the interviewer should then ask 'Do you do "x" now?' and 'Would you like to be able to do "x" now?' Even if the client answers 'No' to 'Do you do "x" now?', the interviewer should still proceed to 'Would you like to be able to do "x" now?'

e.g. Interviewer: Do you like swimming?
     Client: Yes.
     Interviewer: Do you go swimming now?
     Client: No.
     Interviewer: Would you like to be able to go swimming?
     Client: Yes.

2. Between sections (c) and (d) in question 7, insert:
   YES NO *Or are you learning at home?*
   YES NO With someone teaching you? Who? ....
   YES NO Correspondence course?
   YES NO Cassette teaching?
   YES NO Home computer?
   YES NO Some other kind of learning? Describe it ....

3. Insert the following after 8 (c):
   YES NO *Are you attending any training in order to get a job?*
   YES NO Voluntary work?
   YES NO Adult Training Centre?
   YES NO Apprenticeship?
   YES NO Further Education College?
   YES NO Other please specify:

4. Omit 8(d), and replace with:
   'Would you like to go out to work?'

FURTHER READING

For further reading on the use of questionnaires and interviewing techniques with people who have mental handicaps, see:

Flynn, M.C. (1986) Adults who are mentally handicapped as consumers: issues and guidelines for interviewing. *Journal of Mental Deficiency Research*, **30**, 369–377.
Jones, M. (1986) An examination of the lifestyle of residents in a group home. *Australian and New Zealand Journal of Developmental Disabilities*, **12** (22) 133–137.

QUESTIONNAIRE: DAYTIME ACTIVITIES

Introduction

We would like to find out the sorts of daytime activities that you/your client would like to have available outside of you/your client's home.

These daytime activities could include an interest or hobby, learning something new, training for work or work itself.

First I'd like to ask you a few general details:

Client's Name .... :   If this is being filled in by the Support/
                                               :   Key Worker please give the details

Client's Name .... : If this is being filled in by the Support/
: Key Worker please give the details
: below:
Age .... :
Sex .... : Your name ....
Occupation .... :
Address .... : Job ....
(at present) ....:
.... :
Address .... : Address (best contacted at)
(Future) ....:
.... :   ....

Tel. No. .... : Tel. No. ....

Date of completing this form ....

(Circle the answer to the following questions)

1. Mobility
   YES   NO   Do you use public transport?
   YES   NO   Without help?
   YES   NO   Do you climb stairs?
   YES   NO   Without help
   YES   NO   Do you use a wheelchair, walking stick, walking frame, other
                  walking aid? If so, which one do you use?

Thank you. Now we'll go onto the next part.
I'm going to ask you some questions about the things you like doing at the moment, and that you might like to do when you leave hospital.

2. YES   NO   Do you go out?
                If YES where do you go?
                (If NO, go to 3)
   YES   NO   Do you go work?
                If YES, where do you work ....
   YES   NO   Do you go to a centre?
                If YES, which centre do you go to? ....
   YES   NO   Do you go to a class?
                If YES, which class do you go to? ....
   YES   NO   Do you go to somewhere else?
                If YES, where do you go? ....

Could you tell me what you do there?
(Again if no answer, continue)

3. YES   NO   Do you like sport?
                If YES, ask:
                'Do you do "x" at the moment?'
                Would you, like to do "x" when you move out of hospital?'

			At the moment		When you move	
			YES	NO	YES	NO
YES	NO	Walking	:		:	:
YES	NO	Swimming	:		:	:
YES	NO	Horseriding	:		:	
YES	NO	Ball games	:		:	:
YES	NO	Football	:		:	:
YES	NO	Dancing	:		:	:

YES NO   Are there any other sports you like doing? (e.g. yoga, cycling, keep fit)

4. YES NO   *Do you like going out or seeing your friends or relatives?*
If YES, Do you like:

			At the moment		When you move	
			YES	NO	YES	NO
YES	NO	Visiting friends/ relatives	:	:	:	:
YES	NO	Having visitors	:	:	:	:
YES	NO	Going to a cafe or pub	:	:	:	:
YES	NO	Going to a disco	:	:	:	:
YES	NO	Going to a club	:	:	:	:
YES	NO	Singing	:	:	:	:
YES	NO	going on outings	:	:	:	:
YES	NO	Going to a lunch club	:	:	:	:
YES	NO	Going to bingo	:	:	:	:
YES	NO	Going to a cinema	:	:	:	:
YES	NO	Going to concerts	:	:	:	:
YES	NO	Going on holidays	:	:	:	:

YES NO   Are there any other places you like to go? (e.g. going to the theatre)

5. YES NO   *Do you like doing things at home/on the ward*
If YES, Do you like:

			At the moment		When you move	
			YES	NO	YES	NO
YES	NO	Sewing or needlework	:	:	:	:
YES	NO	Knitting	:	:	:	:
YES	NO	Watching TV	:	:	:	:
YES	NO	Listening to the radio	:	:	:	:
YES	NO	Listening to records/tapes	:	:	:	:
YES	NO	Looking after pets	:	:	:	:

			At the moment		When you move	
			YES	NO	YES	NO
YES	NO	Cooking	:		:		:
YES	NO	Reading	:		:		:
YES	NO	Board and	:		:		:
		card games	:		:		:
YES	NO	Gardening	:		:		:

YES   NO   Are there any other things you like doing around the house/ward?
(e.g. fixing things, playing with computers)

6. YES   NO   *Do you like doing arts and crafts?*
If YES, Do you like:

			At the moment		When you move	
			YES	NO	YES	NO
YES	NO	Painting	:		:		:
YES	NO	Pottery	:		:		:
YES	NO	Playing a	:		:		:
		musical				
		instrument	:		:		:

YES   NO   Are there other arts and crafts you like doing
(e.g. photography, weaving?)

Right, we've talked about your hobbies . . . . . .

7. YES   NO   *Are you attending a college or centre?*
If YES, is it:

(a) YES   NO   *an Adult Education Institute?* Which one? . . . . .
  YES   NO   is it a 'special' class?
  YES   NO   an 'Integrated' class?
  YES   NO   Would you like to keep going to classes when you leave hospital?

(b) YES   NO   *or Adult Training Centre?* Which one? . . . . . .
  YES   NO   Would you like to keep going there when you leave hospital?

(c) YES   NO   *or somewhere else?* Where? . . . . . .
  YES   NO   Would you like to keep going there when you leave hospital?

(d) *At the centre/class, are you learning things to help you are home?*
  YES   NO   How to cook healthy foods?
  YES   NO   How to look after yourself?
          (e.g. grooming, looking after clothes)
  YES   NO   How to look after a house?
          (e.g. house cleaning, ironing, paying bills)
  YES   NO   Are there other things you are learning to do?
          What are they? ....
  YES   NO   *Would you like to keep on learning these things when you leave hospital?*

8.
(a) YES   NO   *Do you have a job at present?* What do you do? ....
(b) YES   NO   *Have you had a job in the past?* If so, what did you do? .....
      ....

(c) *If you have or had a job how did you get it?*
    YES   NO   Someone found you a job
    YES   NO   Advertisement in a paper
    YES   NO   Employment agency
    YES   NO   Word of mouth
(d) YES   NO   *Would you like to get a job when you leave hospital?*
                    (if NO, go to question 9)
                    If YES:
(e) *Would you like full-time or part-time work?* ....
(f) *What kind of work would you like?* ....
....
(g) *Why would you like to work?*
    YES   NO   To meet people
    YES   NO   To earn money
    YES   NO   To get out
    YES   NO   Are there any other reasons why you'd like to work? What are they?
    YES   NO   Would you be prepared to be involved in some training to get a job?

9. *When you go out would you like to be:*
    YES   NO   On your own?
    YES   NO   On your own in a small group?
    YES   NO   On your own in a large group?
    YES   NO   With someone you know?
    YES   NO   With someone you know in a small group?
    YES   NO   With someone you know in a large group?

10. *Of the things you've said, which do you think you would like to try first?*

11. *Is there any activity that you specifically don't want to do?*

12. *Are there any other things you would like to say?*

Thank you for taking time to answer all the questions.

Appendix 3

Some information about Habinteg in Southwark

The development at Simms Road, St James, Bermondsey, London SE1

Client
  Habinteg Housing Association Ltd.
  6 Dukes Mews
  London W1M IRB
  Tel. O1 935 6931

Structural Engineer
  Alan Baxter and Associates
  14–16 Cowcross Street
  London EC1M 6DR
  Tel. 01-250 1555

Architects
  Design Research Unit
  Architects and Designers
  94 Lower Marsh
  London SE1 7AB
  Tel. 01 633 9711

Quantity Surveyor
  PFP Project & Management
  Consultants
  5 Manchester Square
  London W1A 1AU
  Tel. 01 486 4331

Services Engineer
   James R. Briggs & Associates
   Tollington House
   598 Holloway Road
   London N19 3PH
   Tel. 01 272 8979

References

Aeschleman, S.R. and Schladenhauffen, J. (1984) Acquisition, generalisation and maintenance of grocery shopping skills by severely mentally retarded adolescents. *Applied Research in Mental Retardation*, **5**, 245–58.

Aeschleman, S.R. and Gedig, K.S. (1985) Teaching bank skills to mildly retarded adolescents. *Applied Research in Mental Retardation*, **6**, 449–64.

Allen, P. (1983) Training direct care staff, in *An Ordinary Life: Issues and Strategies for Training Staff for Community Mental Handicap Services* (ed. A. Shearer) King's Fund, London, pp.35–42.

Allen, D. (1989) The effects of deinstitutionalization on people with mental handicaps: a review, *Mental Handicap Research*, **2** (1), 18–37.

Allen, S. and Willet, N. (1986) Improving the communication skills of mentally handicapped adults. *British Journal of Occupational Therapy*, **49** (4), 130–32.

Andrews, B. (1983) Further education for intellectually handicapped students. *Australian Rehabilitation Review*, **7** (4), 19–24.

Andrews, R.J., Elkins, J. and Berry, P.B. (1983) *Evaluation Standards and Accreditation of Government-subsidised Services for Handicapped People: Schonell Evaluation and Accreditation Procedure*, Department of Social Security, Canberra.

Anstice, B. and Bowden, R. (1985) The role of the occupational therapist, in *Mental Handicap: a Multidisciplinary Approach* (eds M. Craft, J. Bicknell and S. Hollins) Baillière Tindall, London, pp.354–64.

Armstrong, J. and Rennie, J. (1986) We can use computers too! The setting up of a project for mentally handicapped residents. *British Journal of Occupational Therapy*, **49** (9), 297–300.

Astell-Burt, C. (1981) *Puppetry for Mentally Handicapped People*, Souvenir Press, London.

Astrachan, M. (1985) Group psychotherapy with mentally retarded female adolescents and adults. *American Journal of Mental Deficiency*, **60**, 152, 156.

Atkinson, D. (1988) Moving from hospital to the community: factors influencing the lifestyles of people with mental handicaps. *Mental Handicap*, **16** (1), 8–11.

Averill, L., Lee, H. and Felce, D. (1989) *A guide to training resources in mental handicap*, BIMH/CCETSW, Kidderminster.

Axline, V. (1969) *Play Therapy*, Ballantine, New York.

Ayres, A.J. (1972) *Sensory Integration and Learning Disorders*, Western Psychological Services, Los Angeles.

Ayres, A.J. (1980) *Sensory Integration and the Child*, Western Psychological Services, Los Angeles.

Balbernie, R. (1985a) Psychotherapy with a mentally handicapped boy. *Journal of Child Psychotherapy*, **11** (2), 65–76.

Balbernie, (1985b) Psychotherapy with an ESN headbanger. *British Journal of Psychotherapy*, **1** (4), 266–73.

Balbernie, R. (1987) Psychotherapy: a resource for use with people with mental handicaps. *Mental Handicap* **15** (1), 16–18.

Baldwin, V.L., Fredericks, H.D. and Brodsky, G. cited in Lederman, E. (1984) *Occupational Therapy in Mental Retardation*, Charles C. Thomas, Springfield, Illinois, p. 372.

Balla, D.A. (1976) Relationship of institution size to quality of care: a review of the literature. *American Journal of Mental Deficiency* **81** (2), 117–24.

Balla, D., Butterfield, E.C. and Zigler, E. (1974) Effects of institutionalisation on retarded children: a longitudinal, cross institutional investigation. *American Journal of Mental Deficiency*, **78** (5), 530–49.

Balla, D.A. and Zigler, E. (1975) Pre-institutional social deprivation responsiveness to social reinforcement and IQ change in institutionalised retarded individuals. *American Journal of Mental Deficiency*, **80** (2), 228–30.

Ballard, K.D., Monk, G., Medcalf, J. *et al.* (1987) Teaching telephone skills in a workshop setting to adults who have intellectual handicaps: two data based case studies. *Australian and New Zealand Journal of Developmental Disabilities* **13** (1), 29–38.

Ballard, R. (1982) Taking the family into account. *Mental Handicap* **10** (3), 75–76.

Baquer, A. (1976) Count and be counted. *Parents Voice*, **26** (3), 11–14.

Baran, F.N. (1972) Group therapy improves mental retardate behaviour. *Hospital and Community Psychiatry*, **23** (1), 7–11.

Barker, P. (1987) *Basic Family Therapy*, Granada, London.

Baroff, G.S. (1980) On size and quality of residential care: a second look. *Mental Retardation*, **18** (3), 113–17.

Bartnik, E. (1981) Deinstitutionalisation and the intellectually handicapped. Part 1: The concept of transition. *Australian Occupational Therapy Journal*, **28** (2), 63–9.

Bartnik, E., Jones G. and Hunter, T. (1981) Deinstitutionalisation and the intellectually handicapped. Part 2: Developing strategies to improve the transition process. *Australian Occupational Therapy Journal*, **28** (3), 111–18.

Barton, R. (1956) *Institutional Neurosis*, Wright, Bristol.

Bates, P. (1980) The effectiveness of interpersonal skills training on the social skill acquisition of moderately and mildly retarded adults. *Journal of Applied Behaviour Analysis*, **13** (2), 237–48.

Behan, S. (1979) A sensori-motor programme for profoundly and severely multiply handicapped children in an institutional setting. *Australian Occupational Therapy Journal*, **26** (4), 178–81.

Bellamy, G.T., Horner, R.H. and Inman, D.P. (1979) *Vocational Habilitation of Severely Retarded Adults – a Direct Service Technology*, University Park Press, Baltimore.

Bender, M. (1986) Crisis of closure. *Health and Social Services Journal*, April 17, 524–5.

Bender, M., Valletutti, P.J. and Bender, R. (1976) *Teaching the Moderately and Severely Handicapped – Curriculum Objectives, Strategies and Activities: I. Behaviour, Self Care and Gross and Fine Motor Skills. II. Communication, Socialisation, Safety and Leisure-time Skills. III. Functional Academics for the Mildly and Moderately Handicapped*, University Park Press, Baltimore.

Bennet, G.K. (1965) *Hand Tool Dexterity Test*, The Psychological Corporation, New York.

Benson, B.A. (1985) Behaviour disorder and mental retardation: associations with age, sex and level of functioning in an out patient clinic sample. *Applied Research in Mental Retardation*, **6**, 79–85.

Bentovim, A., Gorell Barnes, G. and Cooklin, A. (eds) (1982a) *Family Therapy: Volume 1*, Academic Press, London.

Bentovim, A., Gorell Barnes, G. and Cooklin A. (eds) (1982b) *Family Therapy: Volume 2*, Academic Press, London.

Berdiansky, H.A. and Parker, R. (1977) Establishing a group home for the adult mentally retarded in North Carolina. *Mental Retardation*, **15** (4), 8–11.

Berger, M. (1983) Predictable tasks in therapy with families of handicapped persons, in *Questions and Answers in Family Therapy, Volume 2*. (ed. A.S. Gurman) Brunner-Mazel, New York, pp. 82–7.

Bergreen, M. (1971) A study of mental health of near relatives of twenty multi-handicapped children. *Acta Paediatrica Scandinavica*, Suppl. **215** (1), 1–24.

Berne, E. (1964) *Games People Play*, Penguin, London.

Berry, P. (1985) Evaluation of residential provision, (eds M. Craft, J. Bicknell and S. Hollins) *Mental Handicap: a Multidisciplinary Approach* Baillière Tindall, London, pp.24–32.

Heal, B.W. (1982) Resident release patterns in a national sample of public residential facilities. *American Journal of Mental Deficiency* **87**, 130–140.

Bettison, S., Davison, D., Taylor, P. and Fox, B. (1976) The long-term effects of a toilet training programme for the retarded: a pilot study. *Australian Journal of Mental Retardation*, **4**, 28–35.

Bicknell, D.J. (1983) Living with a mentally handicapped member of the family. *Postgraduate Medical Journal*, **58** (1), 3–11.

Birenbaum, A. and Re, M. (1979) Resettling mentally retarded adults in the community–almost 4 years later. *American Journal of Mental Deficiency*, **83** (4), 323–9.

Bjaanes, A. and Butler, E. (1974) Environmental variations in community care facilities for mentally retarded persons. *American Journal of Mental Deficiency*, **78** (4), 429–39.

Black, D. (1982) Handicap and family therapy, in *Family Therapy: Volume 2* (eds. A. Bentovim, G. Gorell Barnes and A. Cooklin) Academic Press, London, pp.417–39.

Bluma, S., Shearer, M., Frohman, A. and Hilliard, J. (1976) *Portage Guide to Early Education*, NFER-Nelson, Windsor.

Blundy, C. and Prevezer, K. (1986) the occupational therapist as a member of the community mental handicap team. *British Journal of Occupational Therapy*, **49** (4), 107–10.

Bobath, B. (1978) *Adult Hemiplegia: Evaluation and Treatment*, Heinemann Medical, London.

Hallenbeck, P.N., Behrens, D.A. (1966) Clothing problems of the retarded. *Mental Retardation* **5** (1), 21–5.

Bodenham, J. (1983) Freedom of choice for the mentally handicapped. *British Journal of Occupational Therapy*, **46** (12), 356–8.

Booth, T., Phillips, D., Berry, S., Jones, D., Lee, M., Matthews, J., Melotte, C., Pritlove, J. (1989) Home from home: a survey of independent living schemes for people with mental handicaps. *Mental Handicap Research*, **2** (2), 152–65.

Borum, B. (1987) Asian handicaps. *New Society*, 20 March, 22–23.

Bouras, N. (1986) *Psychiatric and Emotional Disorders in Mentally Handicapped People*, unpublished paper, Department of Psychiatry, Guy's Medical School.

Bouras, N., Drummond, K., Brooks, D., Laws, M. (1988) *Mental Handicap and Mental Health: a Community Service*, National Unit for Psychiatric Research and Development, London.

Bouras, N., Drummond, K. (1989) *Community Psychiatric Service in Mental Handicap: Six Years of Experience*, National Unit for Psychiatric Research and Development, London.

Bowden, R. (1985) Organising community services. *Second European Congress of Occupational Therapists*, London.

Bradlyn, A.S., Himadi, W.G., Crimmins, D.B. *et al.* (1983) Conversational skills training for retarded adolescents. *Behaviour Therapy*, **14**, 314–25.

Brandes, D. and Phillips, H. (1977) *Gamester's Handbook*, Hutchinson, London.

Bratt, A. and Johnson, R. (1988) Changes in lifestyle for young adults with profound handicaps following discharge from hospital care into a 'second generation' housing project. *Mental Handicap Research*, **1**, 49–74.

British Psychological Society (1984) Evidence to the House of Commons Social Services Committee on Community Care, with special reference to the adult mentally ill and mentally handicapped. *Bulletin of the British Psychological Society*, **37**, 378–80.

Brody, E. (1973) A million procrustean beds. *The Gerontologist*, **14**, 430–5.

Bollier, C., Bender, D., Cyranowski, J. and Moseley-Velletri, C. (1986) A pilot study of job burnouts amongst hospital based occupational therapists. *The Occupational Therapy Journal of Research*, **6** (5), 285–99.

Brough, D. and Hooyveld, L. (1978) The role of the community O.T. in a multiprofessional psychiatric team. *British Journal of Occupational Therapy*, **41** (6), 196–9.

Brown, L., Shiraga, B., Rogan, P. *et al.* (1985) *The 'Why' Question in Educational Programmes for Students who are Severely Intellectually Disabled*, University of Wisconsin and Madison Metropolitan School District.

Brown, S. (1984) An evaluation of chair bases for use on carpet by children with cerebral palsy. *Australian Occupational Therapy Journal* **31** (4), 152–5.

Brudenell, P. (1986) *The Other Side of Profound Handicap*, Macmillan Education, London.

Bruininks, R.H., Thurlow, M.L., Thurman, K. and Fiorelli, J.A. (1980) Deinstitutionalisation and community services, in *Mental Retardation and Developmental Disabilities No. 11* (ed. J. Wortis) Brunner-Mazel, New York, pp.55–101.

Buckley, P., Karasu, T.B. and Charles, E. (1979) Common mistakes in psychotherapy. *American Journal of Psychiatry*, **136** (12), 1578–80.

Burnett-Beaulieu, S. (1982) Occupational therapy dropouts: escape from the grief process. *Occupational Therapy in Mental Health*, **2** (2), 45–55.

Caldwell, P. (1985) Introducing specialised equipment to the profoundly mentally handicapped person with behaviour disturbance. *British Association of Occupational Therapists Special Interest Group – Mental Handicap*, September Meeting.

Campaign for People with Mental Handicaps (1986) *Self Advocacy Package*, Campaign for People with Mental Handicaps, London.

Campbell, A.C. (1968) Comparisons of family and community contacts of mentally subnormal adults in hospital and local authority hostels. *British Journal of Prevention and Social Medicine* **22** (3), 165–9.

Campbell, D.A. (1975) Project alternative: a therapeutic social group. *Canadian Journal of Occupational Therapy*, **42** (4), 145–9.

Carle, N. (1984) *Key concepts (5) – Citizen Advocacy*, Campaign for People with Mental Handicaps, London.

Carpenter, P.R. and Axson, D.M. (1989) The Myrtle Cottage project: testing resettlement groupings. *Mental Handicap*, **17** (3), 94–6.

Carr, J. (1985) The effect on the family, in *Mental Deficiency – the Changing Outlook* (eds A.M. Clarke, A.D.B. Clarke and J.M. Berg) Methuen, London, pp.512–48.

Cassidy, N., Ash, B., Coombs, B. and Bubb, P. (1986) 'So then we will be outsiders': one ressettlement team's experience of assessing and preparing people with a mental handicap for life in the community. *British Journal of Occupational Therapy*, **49** (4), 103–6.

Charrier, G.O. (1972) Cog's ladder: a model of group development. *Advanced Management Journal*, **37** (1), 30–37.

Chia, S.H. (1985) The Bobath approach and its application to occupational therapy for children with cerebral palsy. *British Journal of Occupational Therapy*, **48** (1), 4–7.

Christoff, K.A. and Kelly, J.A. (1983) Social Skills, in *Assessing the Retarded* (eds J.L. Matson and S.E. Breuning) Grune and Stratton, New York, pp. 181–206.

Chu, S.K.H. (1989) The application of contemporary treatment approaches for children with cerebral palsy. *British Journal of Occupational Therapy*, **52** (9), 343–8.

Clarke, D. (1984) *Help, Hospitals and the Handicapped*, Aberdeen University Press, Aberdeen.

Cleland, C.C. (1979) *The Profoundly Mentally Retarded*, Prentice-Hall, New Jersey.

Close, D.W. (1977) Community living for severely and profoundly retarded adults: a group home study. *Education and Training of the Mentally Retarded*, **12**, 256–62.

Close, W., Carpenter, M. and Cibri, S. (1986) An evaluation study of sensory motor therapy for profoundly retarded adults. *Canadian Journal of Occupational Therapy*, **53** (5), 259–64.

Cochran, W.E., Sran, P.K. and Varano, G.A. (1977) The relocation syndrome in mentally retarded individuals. *Mental Retardation*. **15** (2), 10–12.

Coffman, T.L. and Harris, M.C. (1980) Transition shock and adjustments of mentally retarded individuals. *Mental Retardation*, **18** (1), 3–7.

Cole, A. (1989) Group work with people who have a mental handicap – an approach marred by scepticism? *Mental Handicap*, **17** (3), 115–18.

Conacher, G. (ed.) (1986) *Kitchen Sense for Disabled People*, Croom Helm, Dover, New Hampshire.

Copeland, M., Ford, I. and Solon, N. (1976) *Occupational Therapy for Mentally Retarded Children*, University Park Press, Baltimore.

Corbett, J.A. (1979) Psychiatric morbidity and mental retardation in *Psychiatric Illness and Mental Handicap* (eds P. Snaith and F.E. James), Headly Brothers, Ashford, Kent.

Correia, S. (ed.) (1981) A critical self analysis by occupational therapists in the Guy's District. *British Journal of Occupational Therapy*, **44**, (2) 44–7.

Cox, C. (1988) Practical aspects of stress management. *British Journal of Occupational Therapy*, **51** (2), 44–7.

Craik, C. (1988) Stress in occupational therapy: how to cope. *British Journal of Occupational Therapy*, **51** (2), 40–3.

Crawford, J.D. (1987) Individual psychotherapy with the non-vocal patient: a unique application of communication devices. *Rehabilitation Psychology*, **32** (2), 93–8.

Crawford, J.L., Aiello, J.R. and Thompson, D.E. (1979) Deinstitutionalisation and community placement: clinical and environmental factors. *Mental Retardation*, **17** (2), 59–63.

Crawley, J. (1978) The life cycle of the group. *Small Groups Newsletter, Australia* **1** (2), 39–44.

Crawley, J. (1979) The nature of leadership in small groups. *Small Groups Newsletter, Australia* **2** (3).

Critchley, D. (1989) *Occupational Therapy Designed Activities for Clients with Severe Intellectual and Physical Disabilities*, Spastic Society, Melbourne.

Crnic, K.A., Friedrich, W.N. and Greenberg, M.T. (1983) Adaptation of families with mentally retarded children: a model of stress, coping and family etiology. *American Journal of Mental Deficiency*, **88** (2), 125–38.

Cromwell, F.S. (1986) *Computer applications in occupational therapy*, Haworth Press, London.

Crossley, R. and McDonald, A. (1984) *Annie's Coming Out*, Penguin, Melbourne, Australia.

Cummings, R., Emerson, E., Barrett, S., McCool, C., Toogood, A., Hughes, H. (1989) Challenging behaviour and community services 4: Establishing services. *Mental Handicap*, **17** (1), 13–17.

Cunnick, W.R. and Smith, N. (1977) Occupationally related emotional problems. *New York Journal of Medicine*, **77** (11), 1737–41.

Cunningham, C. and Davis, H. (1985) cited in Swain, J. and Eagle, P. (1987) The views of parents and carers: 2. Working with others. *Mental Handicap*, **15** (4), 152–4.

Dalgleish, M. (1986) Family contacts of mentally handicapped adults in different types of residential care. *British Journal of Mental Subnormality*, **31** (1), 114–16.

Davies, L. (1987) *Quality, costs, and an ordinary life: comparing the cost and quality of different residential services for people with mental handicaps.* King's Fund, London.

Davison, H., Saxton K. (1989) 'When are we going to move?' *Mental Handicap*, **17** (3), 92–4.

Dawson, R., Huddleston, S. (1983) The action chair *British Journal of Occupational Therapy* **46** (2), 49–54.

Day, K. (1983) A hospital based psychiatric unit for mentally handicapped adults. *Mental Handicap*, **11**, 137–40.

Day, P.R. (1988) Not an ordinary life. *Mental Handicap*, **16** (1), 4–7.

Day, P.R. (1989) Uncertain future: experiences and expectations of people with mental handicaps of life beyond the hospital and hostel. *Mental Handicap Research*, **2** (2), 166–85.

de Kock, U., Saxby, H., Thomas, M. and Felce, D. (1988) Community and family contact: an evaluation of small community homes for adults with severe and profound mental handicap. *Mental Handicap Research*, 1 (2), 127–40.

De Maars, P.K. (1975) Training adult retardates for private enterprise. *American Journal of Occupational Therapy*, 29 (1), 39–42.

Department of Health and Social Security (1971) *Better Services for the Mentally Handicapped*, HMSO, London.

Department of Youth, Sport and Recreation (1976) *New Games* Dept. Youth, Sport & Recreation, Melbourne.

Development Group for Services to Mentally Handicapped People (1981) *Report to District Management Team, Guy's District*, London.

Dies, R. (1980) Current practice in the training of group psychotherapists. *International Journal of Group Psychotherapy*, 30 (2), 169–85.

DiMichael, S.G. and Terwillinger, W.B. (1953) 'Counsellors' activities in the vocational rehabilitation of the mentally retarded. *Journal of Clinical Psychology*, 9, 99–106.

Doll, P. (1953) Cited in Symington, N. (1981) The psychotherapy of a subnormal patient. *British Journal of Medical Psychology*, 54, 198.

Donges, G.S. (1982) *Policy Making for the Mentally Handicapped*, Gower, Aldershot.

Donkersley, M., Thorpe, M. (1989) Video assisted learning for adults with mental handicaps. *Mental Handicap*, 17 (2), 74–77.

Dudman, V. and Shaw, H. (1987) Home assessment and housing adaptations, in *Occupational therapy in the community* (ed. E. Bumphrey), Woodhead-Faulkner, Cambridge, pp.108–135.

Dunn, F., Ross, B. and Patterson, R. (1984) *Citizen Advocacy Project Development*, unpublished paper, Mental Retardation Division, Melbourne.

Dunn, J.M. and Moorehouse, J.W. (1980) *A Data Based Gymnasium: a Systematic Approach to Physical Education for the Handicapped*, Instructional Development Corporation, Monomonth, Oregon, pp.5–13.

Durrant, P. (1985) Glenda's story. *Community Care*, April 4, 17–18.

Dy, E.B., Strain, P., Fullerton, A. and Stowitschek, J. (1981) Training institutionalised elderly mentally retarded persons as intervention agents for socially isolate peers. *Analysis & Intervention in Developmental Disabilities*, 2, 199–215.

Dyson, S. (1987) *Mental handicap: dilemmas of parent–professional relations*, Croom Helm, London.

Eakin, P. (1989a) Assessments of activities of daily living: a critical review. *British Journal of Occupational Therapy*, 52 (1), 11–15.

Eakin, P. (1989b) Problems with assessments of activities of daily living. *British Journal of Occupational Therapy*, 52 (2), 50–54.

Eaton, L.F., Mendascino, F.J. (1982) Psychiatric disorders in the retarded: problems and challenges. *American Journal of Psychiatry*, 139, 1297–303.

Eden, S. (1987) Ethnic groups, in *Occupational Therapy in the Community* (ed. E. Bumphrey), Woodhead-Faulkner, Cambridge, pp.223-33.

Elkins, J., Andrews, R.J., Berry, P.B. Wells, B. (1980) *The Future of Services for Handicapped Persons in Australia*, Fred & Eleanor Schonell Education and Research Centre, St Lucia, Queensland.

Ellis, N.R. (1983) Toilet training the severely defective patient: an S-R enforcement analysis. *American Journal of Mental Deficiency*, **68**, 98–103.

Ellis, N.R., Balla, D., Estes, O. *et al* (1981) Common sense in the habilitation of mentally retarded persons: a reply to Menolascino and McGee. *Mental Retardation*, **19**, 221–6.

Ellis, N.R., Deacon, J.R., Harris, L.A. *et al.* (1982) Learning, memory and transfer in profoundly, severely and moderately retarded persons. *American Journal of Mental Deficiency*, **87**, 186–96.

Emerson, E., Toogood, A., Mansell, J. *et al.* (1988) Challenging behaviour and community services: 2. Who are the people who challenge services? *Mental Handicap*, **16** (1), 16–19.

Englehardt, H.T. (1977) Defining occupational therapy; the meaning of therapy and virtues of occupation. *American Journal of Occupational Therapy*, **31** (10), 666–8.

Evans, G., Beyer, S., Todd, S. and Blunden, R. (1986) Planning for the All-Wales Strategy. *Mental Handicap*, **14** (3), 108–10.

Evans, G., Todd, S., Blunden, R. *et al.* (1987) Evaluating the impact of a move to ordinary housing. *British Journal of Mental Subnormality* **32** (1), 10–18.

Eyman, R.K. (1976) Trends in the development of the profoundly retarded In *Research on the Profoundly Retarded: Second Annual Conference Proceedings.* (ed. C.C. Cleland) Western Research Conference, Austin, Texas, pp.15–21.

Eyman, R.K. and Call, T. (1977) Maladaptive behaviour and community placement of mentally retarded persons. *American Journal of Mental Deficiency*, **82** (2), 137–44.

Eyman, R.K., Demaine, G.L. and Lei, T. (1979) Relationship between community environments and resident changes in adaptive behaviour: a path model. *American Journal of Mental Deficiency*, **83** (4), 330–8.

Farber, B. (1959a) cited in Crnic, K.A., Friedrich, W. N. and Greenberg, M.T. (1983) Adaptation of families with mentally retarded children: a model of stress, coping and family etiology. *American Journal of Mental Deficiency*, **88** (2), 125–38.

Farber, B. (1959b) cited in Ferrari, M. (1984) Chronic illness: psychosocial effects on siblings – I. Chronically ill boys. *Journal of Child Psychology and Psychiatry*, **25** (3), 459–76.

Farber, B. (1960) cited in Crnic, K.A., Friedrich, W.N. and Greenberg, M.T. (1983) Adaptation of families with mentally retarded children: a model of stress, coping and family etiology. *American Journal of Mental Deficiency*, **88** (2), 125–38.

Farber, B. (1968) *Mental Retardation: its Social Context and Social Consequences*, Houghton Mifflin, Boston.

Farber, B. (1970) cited in Crnic, K.A., Friedrich, W.N. and Greenberg, M.T. (1983) Adaptation of families with mentally retarded children: a model of stress, coping and family etiology. *American Journal of Mental Deficiency*, **88** (2), 125–38.

Farber, S. (1974) *Sensori-motor Evaluation and Treatment Procedures for Allied Health Personnel*, The Indiana University Foundation, Indianapolis.

Favell, J.E. (1973) Reduction of stereotypes by reinforcement of toy play. *Mental Retardation*, **11** (1), 21–23.

Favell, J.E., Favell, J.E. and McGinsey, J.F. (1978) Relative effectiveness and efficiency of group individual training of severely retarded persons. *American Journal of Mental Deficiency*, **83**, 104–9.

Felce, D. (1981) The capital costs of alternative residential facilities for mentally handicapped people. *British Journal of Psychiatry*, **139**, 230–7.

Felce, D. (1986) Accommodating adults with severe and profound mental handicaps: comparative revenue costs. *Mental Handicap*, **14** (3), 104–7.

Felce, D., Jenkins, J., deKock, U. and Mansell, J. (1986) *The Beereweeke Skill Teaching System and Goals Setting Checklist for Adults*, NFER-Nelson, Windsor.

Felce, D., Jenkins, J., Mansell, J. *et al.* (1982) *Staff Induction Training*, University of Southampton, Health Care Evaluation Team.

Felce, D. and Toogood, A. (1988) *Close to Home*, British Institute of Mental Handicap, Kidderminster.

Ferrari, M. (1984) Chronic illness: psychosocial effects on siblings – I. Chronically ill boys. *Journal of Child Psychology and Psychiatry*, **25** (3), 459–76.

Fewtrell, W.D. (1973) A way of toilet training retarded children. *Apex* **1** (Sept.), 26–7.

Fidura, J.G., Linsey, E.R. and Walker, G.R. (1987) A special behaviour unit for treatment of behaviour problems of persons who are mentally retarded. *Mental Retardation*, **25** (2), 107–11.

Fielding, J. (1982) The Scapegoat, *Course in Group Interactions, Mental Health Commission of Victoria, 1982*.

Fielding, J.M. (1974) Problems of evaluative research into group psychotherapy outcome. *Australian and New Zealand Journal of Psychiatry*, **8** (2), 97–102.

Fielding, J.M. (1975) A technique for measuring outcome in group psychotherapy. *British Journal of Medical Psychology*, **48**, 189–98.

Finnie, N.R. (1974) *Handling the Young Cerebral Palsied Child at Home* Heinemann Medical, London.

Finnie, N.R. (1978) Chaining strategies for teaching sequenced motor tasks to mentally retarded adults. *American Journal of Occupational Therapy*, **32** (1), 385–9,

Firth, H. (1983) Training support staff in *An Ordinary Life: Issues and Strategies for Training Staff for Community Mental Handicap Services* (ed. A. Shearer), King's Fund Centre, London, pp.43–49.

Fleming, W. (1984) Brook Drive Project, *AMPH Conference, Guildford*.

Flynn, M.C. (1986) Adults who are mentally handicapped as consumers: issues and guidelines for interviewing. *Journal of Mental Deficiency Research*, **30**, 369–77.

Flynn, M. and Saleem, J.K. (1986) Adults who are mentally handicapped and living with their parents: satisfaction and perceptions regarding their lives and circumstances. *Journal of Mental Deficiency Research*, **30** (4), 379–87.

Foxx, R.M. and Azrin, N.H. (1973) *Toilet Training the Retarded: a Rapid Programme for Day and Nightime Independent Toileting*, Research Press, Champaign, Illinois.

Foxx, R.M. and Dufrense, D. (1984) 'Harry': the use of physical restraint as a reinforcer, time out from restraint and fading restraint in treating a self-injurious man. *Analysis and Intervention in Developmental Disabilities*, **4**, 1–13.

Foxx, R.M., McMorrow, M.J. and Schloss, C.N. (1983) Stacking the deck: teaching social skills to retarded adults with a modified table game. *Journal of Applied Behaviour Analysis*, **16** (2), 157–70.

Freedman, D. (1988a) Assessing the service needs of people with mental handicaps: the Jay Project phase 1. *Mental Handicap*, **16** (1), 32–35.

Freedman, D. (1988b) Assessing the service needs of people with mental handicaps: method used in the Jay Project. *Mental Handicap*, **16** (2), 80–83.

Freeman, R.D., Mallin, S.F. and Hastings, J.O., (1975) Psychosocial problems of deaf children and their families: a comparative study. *American Annals of the Deaf*, **120**, 391–405.

Freudenberger, H. and Richelson, C. (1980) *Burnout*, Arrow, London.

Friedrich, W.N. and Friedrich, W.L. (1981) Comparison of psychosocial assets of parents with a handicapped child and their normal controls. *American Journal of Mental Deficiency*, **85** (5), 551–3.

Fullerton, M. (1986) Back to base *New Society* 22 August, p.13.

Gath, A. (1974) Siblings reactions to mental handicap: a comparison of the brothers and sisters of mongol children. *Journal of Child Psychology and Psychiatry*, **15** (2), 187–98.

Gath, A. and Gumley, O. (1987) Retarded children and their siblings. *Journal of Child Psychology and Psychiatry*, **28** (5), 715–30.

Gathercole, C.E. (1981a) *Residential Alternatives for Adults who are Mentally Handicapped*, British Institute of Mental Handicap, Kidderminster.

Gathercole, C.E. (1981b) *Ameliorating Transition Shock*, unpublished paper, Lancashire Area Health Authority.

Gaze, H. (1985) Countdown to closure. *Nursing Times*, **81** (21), 18–19.

Goffman, E. (1961) *Asylum: Essays on the Social Situation of Mental Patients and other Inmates*, Penguin, London.

Gorell Barnes, G. (1985) Systems theory and family therapy, in *Child and Adolescent Psychiatry* (ed. M. Rutter and L. Hersov), Blackwell Scientific Publications, Oxford, pp. 216–29.

Gostin, L.O. (1985) The law relating to mental handicap in England and Wales, in *Mental Handicap: a Multidisciplinary Approach* (eds M. Craft, J. Bicknell and S. Hollins), Baillière Tindall, London, pp. 58–72.

Goven, P., Faber, T., Prins, S. and Mangold, B. (1984) *The Use of Sensory Stimulation in Teaching Mentally Impaired Students*, Charles C. Thomas, Springfield, Illinois.

Gow, L. (1988) Integration in Australia. *European Journal of Special Needs Education*, **3** (1), 1–12.

Griffiths, M., Wyatt, J. and Hersov, J. (1985) Further education, adult education and self advocacy, in *Mental Handicap: a Multidisciplinary Approach*. (eds M. Craft, J. Bicknell and S. Hollins), Baillière Tindall, London, pp. 271–7.

Gunzberg, H.C. (1974) Psychotherapy, in *Mental Deficiency: the Changing Outlook* (eds A.M. Clarke and A.D.B. Clarke), Methuen, London, pp. 709–28.

Gunzberg, H.C. (1976) *Progress Assessment Chart of Social and Personal Development*, SEFA Ltd, England.

Haley, J. (1973) *Uncommon Therapy: the Psychiatric Techniques of Milton J. Erickson MD*, W.W. Norton, New York.

Hallenbeck, P.N., Behrens, D.A. (1966) Clothing problems of the retarded *Mental Retardation* **5** (1), 21–5.

Halliday, S. (1987) Parental attitudes to the community care of mentally handicapped children, before and after they move into the community. *British Journal of Mental Subnormality,* **32** (1), 43–9.

Halliday, S. and Potts, M. (1987) Moving into the community: Views from the staff involved in the causes and effects of delays in one move. *British Journal of Mental Subnormality,* **32** (1), 31–41.

Halpern, L.F., Andrasik, F. (1986) The immediate and long term effectiveness of over corrections in treating self-injurious behaviour in a mentally retarded adult. *Applied Research in Mental Retardation* **7**, 59–65.

Halpern, A.S. and Berard, W.R. (1974) Counselling the mentally retarded: a review for practice, in *Mental Retardation Rehabilation and Counselling* (ed. P. Browning), Charles C. Thomas, Springfield, Illinois.

Halpern, A.S., Close, D.W. and Nelson, D.J. (1986) *On my Own-the Impact of Semi-independent Living Programmes for Adults with Mental Retardation,* Paul Brookes, London.

Hamilton, J., Stephens, L., Allen, P. (1967) controlling aggressive and destructive behaviour in severely retarded institutionalised residents. *American Journal of Mental Deficiency* **71**, 852–6

Hargreaves, J. (1986) *Cookery for Handicapped People,* Souvenir Press, London.

Harris, J.M., Veit, S.W., Allen G.J. and Chinsky J.M. (1974) Aide-resident ratio and ward population density as mediators of social interaction. *American Journal of Mental Deficiency,* **79** (3), 320–26.

Harrison, W., Lecrone, H., Temerlin, M.K. and Trousdale, W.W. (1966) The effect of music and exercise upon the self-help skills of non-verbal retardates. *American Journal of Mental Deficiency,* **71**, 279–82.

Harvey, F. (1966) A review of the assessment of people with a mental handicap: some important consideration. *British Journal of Occupational Therapy,* **49** (4), 119–21.

Heaton-Ward, A. (1976) Psychosis in mental handicap. *British Journal of Psychiatry,* **130**, 525–33.

Heaton-Ward, W.A. and Willey, Y. (1984) *Mental Handicap,* Wright, Bristol.

Hegarty, J.R. (1987) Staff burnout: a single case study. *Mental Handicap,* **15** (3), 93–5.

Heginbotham, C. (1980) Housing choice for mentally handicapped people. *Design for Special Needs,* **23**, 11–13.

Heginbotham, C. (1981) *Housing Projects for Mentally Handicapped People,* CEH, London.

Heller, T. (1978) Group decision making by mentally retarded adults. *American Journal of Mental Deficiency,* **82** (5), 480–486.

Heller, T. (1982) The effects of involuntary residential relocation: a review. *American Journal of Community Psychology* **10** (4), 471–92.

Hemming, H., Lavender, T. and Pill, R. (1981) Quality of life of mentally retarded adults transferred from large institutions to new small units. *American Journal of Mental Deficiency* **86** (2), 157–69.

Heron, A. (1982) *Better Services for the Mentally Handicapped: Lessons from the Sheffield Evaluation Studies,* King's Fund Project Paper 34, London.

Herr, S.S. (1978), cited in Bruininks, R. H., Thurlow, M.L., Thurman, S.K. and Fiorelli, J.S. (1980) Deinstitutionalisation and community services, in *Mental Retardation and Developmental Disabilities* (ed. J. Wortis), Brunner-Mazel, New York, pp.78–9.

Heyde, G.C. (1966) *Modular Arrangement of Predetermined Time Standards (MODAPTS)*, The Australian Association of Predetermined Time Standards and Research, New South Wales.

Hodgetts, D. (1986) A psychotherapy group with people with mental handicaps. *Mental Handicap*, **14** (3), 121–23.

Hoffman, L. (1981) *Foundations of Family Therapy*, Basic Books, New York.

Hogg, J., Sebba, J. (1986a) *Profound Retardation and Multiple Impairment Volume 1: Development*. Croom Helm, London.

Hogg, J., Sebba, J. (1986b) *Profound Retardation and Multiple Impairment Volume 2: Education and Therapy*. Croom Helm, London.

Hollins, S. (1985) Families and handicap, in *Mental Handicap: a Multidisciplinary Approach* (eds M. Craft, J. Bicknell and S. Hollins), Baillière Tindall, London, pp.140–6.

Holt, G., Oliver, B. (1989) Reducing stress in mental handicap teams. *Mental Handicap*, **17** (1), 4–5.

Horner, R.D. (1980) The effects of an environmental enrichment programme on the behaviour of institutionalised, profoundly retarded children. *Journal of Applied Behaviour Analysis*, **13**, 473–91.

Howard, A., Beaill, N., Frankish, P., Grimshaw, J., Ball, T. (1989) Psychotherapy in mental handicap with potentially violent people: some thoughts from practitioners. *Mental Handicap*, **17** (2), 54–56.

Human Policy Press (1987) *Self Advocacy Package*, Human Policy Press, New York.

Hume, C. (1984) Transcultural aspects of psychiatric rehabilitation. *British Journal of Occupational Therapy*, **47** (12), 373–4.

Humphreys, S. and Blunden, R. (1987) A collaborative evaluation of an individual plan system. *British Journal of Mental Subnormality*, **32** (1), 19–30.

Humphreys, S., Lowe, K. and Blunden, R. (1984) The use of degree of dependancy scale for describing the characteristics of clients who are mentally handicapped. *British Journal of Mental Subnormality*, **30** (1), 15–23.

Hunt, A. and Smith, A. (1982) 291 Harrow Road *Nursing Times*, Sept. 22, 1595–6.

Ibbotson, J. (1983) A pattern of supervision for community occupational therapists. *British Journal of Occupational Therapy*, **46** (6), 162–3.

Illot, J. (1988) Stress in occupational therapy: how to cope – Letter. *British Journal of Occupational Therapy*, **51** (4), 134.

International Labour Office (1984) *Employment of Disabled Persons*, ILO, Geneva.

Jackson, S.K. and Butler, A.J. (1963) Prediction of successful community placement of institutionalised retardates. *American Journal of Mental Deficiency*, **68** (2), 211–17.

James, D.H. (1986) Psychiatric and behavioural disorders amongst older severely mentally handicapped patients. *Journal of Mental Deficiency Research*, **30**, 341–5.

Jastak, J.F. and King, D.E. (1979) *Wide Range Employment Sample Test (WREST)*, Guidance Associates of Delaware, New Wilmington, Del.

Jenkins, J., Felce, D., Mansell, J. *et al.* (1984) *Beereweeke Goal Setting Checklist for Adults*, NFER-Nelson, Windsor.

Johnson, D. and Wallace, D. (1986) A happy accident. *Community Care*, October 2, pp.24–5.

Johnson, D.W., Marayama, G., Johnson, R.T. *et al.* (1981) Effects of co-operative, competitive and individualistic goal structures on achievement: a meta-analysis. *Psychological Bulletin*, **89**, 97–102.

Johnson, R. and Garrie, C. (1985) The BBC microcomputer for therapy of intellectual impairment following acquired brain damage. *British Journal of Occupational Therapy*, **48** (2), 46–8.

Joint Commission on Accreditation of Hospitals (1973) *Standards for Community Agencies serving Persons with Mental retardation and other Developmental Disabilities*, Joint Commission on Accreditation of Hospitals, Chicago.

Jones, M. (1986) An examination of the lifestyle of the residents of a group home *Australian and New Zealand Journal of Developmental Disabilities*, **12** (2), 133–7.

Kahn, R. (1978) Job burnout – prevention and remedies. *Public Welfare*, **36** (4), 61–63.

Katz, E. (1968) *The Retarded Adult in the Community*, Charles C. Thomas Springfield, Illinois.

Kauffman (1984) cited in Rhoades, C.M., Browning, P.L. and Thornin, E.J. (1986) Self-help advocacy movement: a promising peer-support system for people with mental disabilities. *Rehabilitation Literature*, **47** (1–2), p.4.

Keene, N. and James, H. (1986) Who needs hospital care? *Mental Handicap*, **14** (3), 101–3.

Kelly, J.A. (1982) *Social Skills Training: a Practical Guide for Interventions*, Springer, New York.

Keogh, D.A., Faw, G.D., Whitman, T.L. and Reid, D.H. (1984) Enhancing leisure skills in severely retarded adolescents through a self-instructional treatment package. *Analysis and Intervention in Developmental Disabilities*, **4**, 333–51.

Kesey, K. (1962) *One Flew over the Cuckoo's Nest*, Dominion Press, Melbourne.

Kewish, L. (1979) Occupational therapists in early intervention in the community. *Australian Occupational Therapy Journal*, **26** (3), 129–37.

Kimbrell, D.L., Luckey, R.E., Barbuto, P.F.P., Love, J.G. (1967) Operation dry pants! an intensive training programme for severley and profoundly retarded *Mental Retardation* **5**, 32–6.

King's Fund (1980) *An Ordinary Life: Comprehensive Locally-based Residential Services for Mentally Handicapped People*, King's Fund Centre, London.

King's Fund Working Group (1984) *An Ordinary Working Life – Vocational Services for People with a Mental Handicap*, King's Fund Centre, London.

Kinnell, H. (1987) Community medical care of people with mental handicaps: room for improvement. *Mental Handicap*, **15** (4), 146–51.

Kirby, N. (1986) Have sheltered workshops a future? *Australasian and New Zealand Journal of Developmental Disabilities*, **12** (3), 187–202.

Kitching, N. (1987) Helping people with mental handicaps cope with bereavement. *Mental Handicap*, **15** (2), 60–63.

Klaber, M.M. (1969) The retarded and institutions for the retarded – a preliminary research report, in *Psychological Problems in Mental Deficiency* (eds S.B. Sarason and J. Doris), 4th edn, Harper & Row, New York.

Kleinberg, J. and Galligan, B. (1983) Effects of deinstitutionalisation on adaptive behaviour of mentally retarded adults. *American Journal of Mental Deficiency*, **88** (1), 21–27.

Kochany, L. and Keller, J. (1987) An analysis of evaluation of the failures of severely disabled individuals in competitive employment, in *Competitive Employment: New Horizons for Severely Disabled Individuals* (ed. P. Wehman), Paul H. Brookes, Baltimore, pp.181–98.

Korn, S.J., Chess, S. and Fernandez, P. (1978) The impact of children's physical handicaps on marital quality and family interaction, in *Child Influence on Marital and Family Interaction: a Life Span Development* (eds R.M. Lerner and G.B. Spanier), Academic Press, New York, pp.299–326.

Krupinski, J. and Lippman L. (1984) Multidisciplinary or nondisciplinary: evaluation of staff functioning in a community health centre. *Australian and New Zealand Journal of Psychiatry*, **18** (2), 172–8.

Lamb, R. (1979) Staff burnout in work with long term patients. *Hospital and Community Psychiatry*, **30** (6), 396–8.

Lavigne, J.V. and Ryan, M. (1979) Psychological adjustment of children with chronic illness. *Pediatrics*, **63** (4), 616–27.

Lawson, M.A. (1983) Seating system for the disabled child *British Journal of Occupational Therapy* **46** (10), 301.

Lederman, E.F. (1984) *Occupational Therapy in Mental Retardation*, Charles C. Thomas, Springfield, Illinois.

Leff, R.B. (1974) Teaching the TMR to dial on the telephone. *Mental Retardation*, **12** (4), 12–13.

Levitt, S. (1982) Movement training, in *Profound Mental Handicap* (ed D. Norris) Costello Educational, Tunbridge Wells, pp.65–74.

Leyin, A. (1988) What shall we tell the neighbours? *Mental Handicap* **16** (1), 11–15.

Lindsay, W.D. (1986) Cognitive changes after social skills training with young mildly mentally handicapped adults. *Journal of Mental Deficiency Research*, **30**, 81–8.

Lindsay, W.D. and Kaprowicz, M. (1987) Challenging negative cognitions: developing confidence in adults by means of cognitive behaviour therapy. *Mental Handicap*, **15** (4), 159–62.

Lippman, L. (1976) The public, in *Changing Patterns in Residential Services* (eds R. Kugel and A. Shearer), President's Committee in Mental Retardation, Washington DC.

Livingstone, D., (1987) Hospitals for the mentally handicapped – run down or reform? *Journal of the Royal College of General Practitioners*, **37**, 97–8.

Locker, D., Rao, D. and Weddell, J.M. (1984) Evaluating community care for the mentally handicapped adult: a comparison of hostel, home and hospital care. *Journal of Mental Deficiency Research*, **28** (3), 189–98.

Lockwood, K. and Bourland, G. (1982) Reduction of self-injurious behaviours by reinforcement and toy use. *Mental Retardation*, **20** (4), 169–73.

Lund, J. (1985) The prevalence of psychiatric morbidity in mentally retarded adults. *Acta Psychiatrica Scandinavia*, **72**, 563–70.

Lyons, M. (1985) Paradise lost. . . .paradise regained? Putting the promise of occupational therapy into practice. *Australian Occupational Therapy Journal*, **32** (2), 45–53.

Lyons, M. (1986) Students as buddies: a proposal for smoothing the path towards broader life experience through recreation. *British Journal of Occupational Therapy*, **49** (4), 111–14.

McBrien, J. (1987) The Haytor unit: specialised day care for adults with severe mental handicaps and behaviour problems. *Mental Handicap*, **15** (2), 77–80.

McBrien, J. and Weightman, J. (1980) The effect of room management procedures on the engagement of profoundly retarded children. *British Journal of Mental Subnormality*, **26** (1), 38–46.

McCool, C., Barrett, S., Emerson, E., Toogood, S., Hughes, H., Cummings, R. (1989) Challenging behaviour and community services 5: structuring staff and client activity. *Mental Handicap*, **17** (2), 60–3.

McCord, W.T. (1981) Community residences: the staffing, in *Mental Retardation and Developmental Disabilities vol. 12* (ed. J. Wortis), Brunner-Mazel, New York, pp.111–18.

McCormick, M., Balla, D. and Zigler, E. (1975) Resident care practices in institutions for retarded persons: a cross-institutional, cross-cultural study. *American Journal of Mental Deficiency*, **80** (1), 1–17.

McCracken, A. (1975) Tactile function of educable mentally retarded children. *American Journal of Occupational Therapy*, **29** (1), 397–402.

McDevitt, S.C., Smith, P.M., Schmidt, D.W. and Rosen, M. (1978) The deinstitutionalised citizen: adjustment and quality of life. *Mental Retardation*, **18** (1), 22–24.

McGowen, C. (1986) Moving on. *British Journal of Occupational Therapy*, **49** (4), 114–116.

McGrath, M. (1988) CMHTs in Wales. *Mental Handicap*, **16** (4), 101–4.

McHatton, M., Collins, G. and Brooks. E. (1988) Evaluation in practice: moving from a problem ward to a staffed flat. *Mental Handicap Research*, **1** (2), 141–51.

McHugh, S. and Knowles, B. (1984) A multidisciplinary approach in psychotherapy. *British Journal of Occupational Therapy*, **47** (2), 36–8.

McKay, A. (1976) A model for community integration through leisure planning and activity. *Canadian Journal of Occupational Therapy*, **43** (2), 66–8.

McLoughlin, C.S., Garner, J.B., Callahan, M. (1987) *Getting employed, staying employed: Job development and training for persons with severe handicaps*, Paul H. Brookes, London.

McMichael, J.K. (1971) *Handicap: a Study of Physically Handicapped Children and their Families*, Staples Press, London.

MacLauchlin, M., Dennis, P., Lang, H. *et al.* (1987) Do the professionals understand? *Mental Handicap*, **15** (1), 5–7.

Malan, D.H. (1979) *Individual Psychotherapy and the Science of Psychodynamics*, Butterworths, London.

Mander, B. and Lyon, B. (1988) The use of self-selected activities and social reinforcement in the management of self-injurious behaviour. *Australian Occupational Therapy Journal*, **35** (2), 59–71.

Mannoni, M. (1973) *The Retarded Child and the Mother*, Tavistock, London.

Mansell, J., Felce, D., deKock, U. and Jenkins, J. (1982) Increasing purposeful activity of severley and profoundly mentally handicapped adults. *Behaviour Research and Therapy*, **20**, 593–604.

Mansell, J., Jenkins, J., Felce, D. and deKock, U. (1984) Measuring the activity of severely and profoundly mentally handicapped adults in ordinary housing. *Behaviour Research and Therapy*, **22** (1), 23–9.

Marholin, D., O'Toole, K.M., Touchette, P.E. *et al.* (1979) 'I'll have a Big Mac, large fries, large Coke and apple pie. . . .'or teaching adaptive community skills. *Behaviour Therapy*, **10**, 236–48.

Martin, G.L. (1974) The future of the severely and profoundly retarded: institutionalisation, normalisation, Kinkare foster homes. *Canadian Psychologist*, **15** (3), 228–41.

Martin, J.E., Rusch, F.R., Lagomarcino, T. and Chadsey-Rusch, J. (1986) Comparison between non-handicapped and mentally retarded workers. *Applied Research in Mental Retardation*, **7**, 467–74.

Mathieson, S., Wilson, C., Jordan, P. and Rowlands, C. (1983) Defining tasks: from policies to job descriptions, in *An Ordinary Life: Issues and Strategies for Training Staff for Community Mental Handicap Services* (ed. A. Shearer), King's Fund Centre, London, pp.22–9.

Matson, J.L. (1981) Use of independence training to teach shopping skills to mildly mentally retarded adults. *American Journal of Mental Deficiency*, **86** (2), 178–83.

Matson, J.L. (1984) Psychotherapy with persons who are mentally retarded. *Mental Retardation*, **22** (4), 170–5.

Matson, J. and Gorman-Smith, D. (1986) A review of treatment research for aggressive and disruptive behaviour in the mentally retarded. *Applied Research in Mental Retardation*, **7**, 95–103.

Matson, J.L. and Senatore, V. (1981) A comparison of traditional psychotherapy and social skills training for improving interpersonal functioning of mentally retarded adults. *Behaviour Therapy*, **12**, 369–82.

Matson, J.L. and Stephens, R.M. (1978) Increasing appropriate behaviour of explosive chronic psychiatric patients with a social skills training package. *Behaviour Modification*, **2** (1), 61–76.

Mattson, A. (1972) Long-term physical illness in childhood: a challenge to psychosocial adaptation. *Pediatrics*, **50** (5), 801–11.

Mayeda, T. and Wai, F. (1975) *The Cost of Long-term Developmental Disabilities Care*, University of California, Los Angeles.

Mayou, R. (1987) Burnout. *British Medical Journal*, **295**, 284–5.

Menchetti, B.M., Rusch, F.R. and Owens, P.M. (1983) Vocational training, in *Assessing the Mentally Retarded* (eds J.L. Matson and S.E. Browning), Grune & Stratton, New York, pp. 245–84.

Menolascino, F.J. (1977) *Challenges in Mental Retardation: Progressive Ideology and Success*, Human Sciences, New York.

Menolascino, F.J., Gilson, S.F. and Levitas, A.S. (1986) Issues in the treatment of mentally retarded patients in the community mental health system. *Community Mental Health Journal*, **22** (4), 314–27.

Menolascino, F.J. and McGee, J.J. (1981) The new institutions: last ditch arguments. *Mental Retardation*, **19**, 215–20.

Meyers, N. (1985) Adapting to a new environment: a personal account of the achievements of three people who are mentally handicapped. *Mental Handicap*, **13** (1), 7–8.

Milne J. and Matthews, P. (1979) Advisers to disabled: Job analysis. *British Journal of Occupational Therapy*, **42** (12), 306–7.

Minuchin, S. (1974) *Families and Family therapy*, Harvard University Press, Cambridge, Mass.

Monfils, M.J. and Menolascino, F.J. (1984) Modified individual and group treatment approaches for the mentally retarded-mentally ill, in *Handbook of Mental Illness in the Mentally Retarded* (eds F.J. Menolascino and J.A. Stark), Plenum Press, New York, pp.155–69.

Moore, P. (1988) *Review of Dressing Matters*, Disabled Living Foundation, London.

Mosey, A.C. (1970) *Three Frames of Reference for Mental Health*, Slack, Thorofare.

Moxley, D., Nevil, N. and Edmonson, B. (1980) *Socialisation Games for Mentally Retarded Adolescents and Adults*, Charles C. Thomas, Springfield, Illinois.

Mulick, J.A., Hoyt, P., Rojahn, J. and Schroeder, S.R. (1978) Reduction of a nervous habit in a profoundly retarded youth by increasing toy play. *Journal of Behaviour Therapy and Experimental Psychiatry*, **9**, 381–5.

Munroe, H. (1988) Modes of operation in clinical supervision: how clinical supervisors see themselves. *British Journal of Occupational Therapy*, **51** (10), 338–43.

Murphy, G. and Wilson, G. (1985) *Self-injurious Behaviour*, BIMH, Kidderminster.

National Development Group (1978) *Helping Mentally Handicapped People Leave Hospital*, HMSO, London

National Development Group for the Mentally Handicapped (1980) *Improving the Quality of Services for Mentally Handicapped People: a Checklist of Standards*, NDG, London.

Neef, N.A., Iwata, B.A. and Page, T.J. (1978) Public transport training: in vivo versus classroom instruction. *Journal of Applied Behaviour Analysis*, **11** (3), 331–44.

Newman, J., Donoghue, K. and Rees, C. (1988) Community mental handicap teams: the role of the occupational therapist. *British Journal of Occupational Therapy*, **51** (8), 273–6.

Nihira, K., Foster, R., Shellhans, M. and Leyland, H. (1984) *AAMD Adaptive Behaviour Scale*, American Association of Mental Deficiency, Washington DC.

Nihira, K., Meyers, C.E. and Mink, I.T. (1980) Home environment, family adjustment and the development of mentally retarded children. *Applied Research in Mental Retardation*, **1** (1), 5–24.

NIMROD (1983) *Preliminary Information on Costs*, NIMROD, Cardiff.

NIMROD (1985) *Criteria for Property for NIMROD Houses*, NIMROD, Cardiff.

Norris, D. (1982) *Profound Mental Handicap*, Costello Educational, Tunbridge Wells.

Nosvogel, S. (1984) Psychiatric disorder in adults admitted to a hospital for the mentally handicapped. *British Journal of Mental Subnormality*, **30** (1), 54–8.

O'Brien, J. and Wolfensberger, W. (1977) *Citizen Advocacy Programme Evaluation*, National Institute on Mental Retardation, Toronto.

Office of Health Economics (1986) *Mental Handicap: Partnership in the Community?* Office of Health Economics/Mencap, London.

Oke, L. (ed.) (1986) *Switches: How to Make them*, Spastic Society of Victoria, Melbourne.

O'Neill, J., Brown, M., Gordon, W. and Schonhorn, R. (1985) The impact of deinstitutionalisation on activities and skills of severely/profoundly mentally retarded multiply handicapped adults. *Applied Research in Mental Retardation*, **6**, 361–71.

Oswin, M. (1981) *Bereavement and Mentally Handicapped People*, King's Fund Centre London.

Oswin, M. (1985) Bereavement, in *Mental Handicap: a Multidisciplinary Approach* (eds M. Craft, J. Bicknell and S. Hollins), Baillière Tindall, London, pp. 197–205.

Page, F. (1986) The therapeutic use of puppetry with mentally handicapped people. *British Journal of Occupational Therapy*, **49** (4), 122–25.

Page, T.J., Iwata, B.A. and Neef, N.A. (1976) Teaching pedestrian skills to retarded persons: generalisation from the classroom to the natural environment. *Journal of Applied Behaviour Analysis*, **9**, 433–444.

Paterson, R. (1986) Facilities and provisions, in *Mental Handicap Handbook of Care* (ed. E. Shanley), Churchill-Livingstone, London, pp.77–104.

Peck, C. and Chia, S.W. (1988) *Living Skills for Mentally Handicapped People*, Croom Helm, London.

Peterson, P. and Wikoff, R.L. (1987) Home environment and adjustment in families with handicapped children: a canonical correlation study. *The Occupational Therapy Journal of Research*, **7** (2), 67–82.

Phil, R.O., Spiers, P. (1977) Some personality differences amongst the multidisciplinary team. *Journal of Clinical Psychology*, **33** (1), 269–72.

Piasecky, J.R., Puttinger, J.E. and Rutman, I.D. (1977) *Determining Costs of Community Residential Services for the Psychosocially Disabled*, National Institute of Mental Health, Rockville, Maryland.

Pines, A. and Maslach, C. (1978) Characteristics of staff burnout in the mental health setting. *Hospital and Community Psychiatry*, **29** (4), 233–7.

Plank, M. (1979) *An Enquiry into Joint Planning of Services for Mentally Handicapped People*, CMH, London.

Pless, I.B. and Pinkerton, P. (1975) cited in Ferrari, M. (1984) Chronic illness: psychosocial effects on siblings – I. Chronically ill boys. *Journal of Child Psychology and Psychiatry*, **25** (3), 459–76.

Pollock, L. (1986) The multidisciplinary team, in *Rehabilition in Psychiatry* (eds C. Hume and I. Pullen), Churchill-Livingstone, London, pp.126–48.

Porterfield, J., Blunden, R. and Blewitt, E. (1980) Improving environments for mentally handicapped adults – using prompts and social attention to maintain high group engagement. *Behaviour Modification*, **4** (2), 225–241.

Porterfield, J. and Gathercole, C. (1985) *The Employment of People with Mental Handicap – Progress Towards an Ordinary Working Life* King's Fund Centre, London.

Potton, A. (1980) The occupational therapist in housing. *Design for Special Needs* **21**, 5–7.

Presland, J.L. (1982) *Paths to Mobility in Special Care*, British Institute of Mental Handicap, Kidderminster.

Rappoport, R. (1963) Normal crises, family structure and mental health. *Family Process*, **2** 68–80.

Rawlings, S. (1985a) Lifestyles of severely retarded, non-communicating adults in hospitals and small residential homes *British Journal of Social Work*, **15**, 281–93.

Rawlings, S. (1985b) Behaviour and skills of severely retarded adults in hospitals and small residential homes. *British Journal of Psychiatry*, **146**, 358–66.

Realon, R.E., Favell, J.E., Stirewalt, S.C. and Phillips, J.F. (1986) Teaching severely handicapped persons to provide leisure activities to peers. *Analysis & Intervention Developmental Disabilities*, **6**, 203–19.

Reed, K.L. (1984) *Models of Practice in OT*, Williams & Wilkins, Baltimore.

Reid, A.H. (1972) Psychoses in adult mental defectives: 1. Manic depressive psychosis; 2. Schizophrenia and paranoid psychosis. *British Journal of Psychiatry*, **120**, 205–18.

Reid, A.H. (1983) The psychiatry of mental handicap: a review. *Journal of the Royal Society of Medicine*, **76**, 587–92.

Reid, A.H. (1985) Psychiatry and mental handicap, in *Mental Handicap: a Multidisciplinary Approach* (eds M. Craft, J. Bicknell and S. Hollins Baillière Tindall, London, pp.317–32.

Reitz, A.L. (1984) Teaching community skills to formerly institutionalised adults: eating nutritionally balanced diets. *Analysis and Intervention in Developmental Disabilities*, **4**, 299–312.

Remocker, A.J. and Storch, E.T. (1977) *Action Speaks Louder*, Churchill-Livingstone, Edinburgh.

Revans, R.W. (1975a) Helping each other to help the helpless. Part 1. *Kybernetes*, **4** (2), 149–55.

Revans, R.W. (1975b) Helping each other to help the helpless. Part 2. *Kybernetes* **4** (3), 205–11.

Richman, G.S., Ponticas, Y., Page, T.J. and Epps, S. (1986) Simulation procedures for teaching independent menstrual care to mentally retarded persons. *Applied Research in Mental Retardation*, **7**, 21–35.

Risley, R. and Cuvo, A.J. (1980) Training mentally retarded adults to make emergency telephone calls. *Behaviour Modification*, **4**, (4), 513–25.

Roberts, W. (1982) Preparation of the referral network: the professional and the family, in *Family Therapy Volume 2.* (eds A. Bentovim, G. Gorell Barnes and A. Cooklin), Academic Press, London, pp.159–71.

Rood, M. (1962) The use of sensory receptors to activate, facilitate and inhibit motor response, automatic and somatic, in developmental sequence. In *Approaches to the treatment of patients with neuromuscular dysfunction* (ed. C. Satley) Brown, Iowa, pp.36–7.

Rudie, F. and Riedl, G. (1984) Attitudes of parents/guardians of mentally retarded former state hospital residents toward current community placement. *American Journal of Mental Deficiency*, **89** (3), 295–7.

Russell, O. (1985) The organization of services towards greater cooperation: patterns of support and care, in *Mental Handicap: a Multidisciplinary Approach* (eds M. Craft, J. Bicknell and S. Hollins), Baillière Tindall, London, pp.6–14

Salzberg, C. and Langford, C.A. (1981) Community integration of mentally retarded adults through leisure activity. *Mental Retardation*, **19**, 127–31.

Sang, B. and O'Brien, J. (1984) *Advocacy – the UK & American Experiences* King's Fund Publication, London.

Sarber, R.E. and Cuvo, A.J. (1983) Teaching nutritional meal planning to developmentally disabled clients. *Behaviour Modification*, **7** (4), 503–30.

Sarber, R.E., Halasz, M.M., Messmer, M.C. *et al.* (1983) Teaching menu planning and grocery shopping skills to a mentally retarded mother. *Mental Retardation*, **21** (3), 101–6.

Saunders, P. (1980) The use of micro-computers in the teaching of the mentally handicapped. *Apex*, **8**, 87–9.

Saxby, H., Thomas, M., Felce, D. and deKock, U. (1986) The use of shops, cafes and public houses by severely and profoundly mentally handicapped adults. *British Journal of Mental Subnormality*, **32**, 69–81.

Schalock, R.L. (1981) *Mid-Nebraska Vocational Training Screening Test*, Mid-Nebraska Mental Retardation Services, Hastings, NE.

Schalock, R.L. and Gadwood, L.L. (1980) *Mid-Nebraska Community Living Skills Screening Test*, Mid-Nebraska Mental Retardation Services, Hastings, NE.

Schalock, R.L. and Harper, R.S. (1978) Placement from community based mental retardation programs: how well do clients do? *American Journal of Mental Deficiency*, **83**, 240–7.

Schalock, R.L. and Lilley, M.A. (1986) Placement from community based mental retardation programmes: how well do clients do after 8 to 10 years? *American Journal of Mental Deficiency*, **90** (6), 669–76.

Schalock, R.L., Ross, B.E. and Ross, I. (1976) *Mid-Nebraska Basic Skills Screening Test*, Mid-Nebraska Mental Retardation Services, Hastings, NE.

Schlesinger, H. and Whelan, E. (1979) *Industry and Effort – a Study of Work Centres in England, Wales & Northern Ireland for Severely Disabled Adults*. The Spastics Society/Heinemann Medical, London.

Scholem, A. and Perlman, B. (1979) The forgotten staff: who cares for the care givers? *Administration in Mental Health*, **6** (1), 21–31.

Schroeder, S.R. and Henes, C. (1976) *An Evaluation of the Effectiveness of Group Homes in the North Central Region of North Carolina, 1974–1975*, Final Grant Report on Contract no. 75A12 to North Carolina Division of Mental Health Research.

Seeger, B.R., Faulkner, P., Caudrey, P.J., (1982) Seating positions and hand functions in Cerebral palsy *Australian Occupational Therapy Journal*, **29** (4), 147–52.

Selan, B.H. (1976) Psychotherapy with the developmentally disabled. *Health Social Work*, **1**, 73–85.

Selvini Palazzoli, M. (ed.) (1978) *Paradox and Counter Paradox*, Jason Aronson, New York.

SETHRA (1987) *Outcomes*, Outset, Bexhill-on-Sea.

Shapiro, A. (1974) Fact and fiction in the care of the mentally handicapped. *British Journal of Psychiatry*, **125**, 286–92.

Shearer, A. (1986) *Building Community with People with Mental Handicaps, their Families and Friends*, Campaign for People with Mental Handicap/King's Fund, London.

Sheppard, J.L., Pollock., J.M., Rayment, S.M. (1983) *Catch Project Social Skills Kit*, Cumberland College of Health Sciences, Sydney.

Silverman, W.P., Silver, E.J., Sersen, E.A. *et al.* (1986) Factors related to adaptive behaviour changes among profoundly mentally retarded, physically disabled persons. *American Journal of Mental Deficiency*, **90** (6), 651–8.

Simon, G.B. (1981) *Local Services for Mentally Handicapped People*, British Institute of Mental Handicap, Kidderminster.

Sinason, V. (1986) Secondary mental handicap and its relationship to trauma. *Psychoanalytic Psychotherapy*, **2** (2), 131–54.

Sinick, D. (1962) cited in Menchetti, B.M., Rusch, F.R. and Owens, D.M. (1983) Vocational training, in *Assessing the Mentally Retarded* (eds J.L. Matson and S.E. Breuning), Grune & Stratton, New York, pp.245–84.

Sireling, L. (1986) Depression in mentally handicapped patients: diagnostic and endocrine evaluation. *British Journal of Psychiatry*, **149**, 274–8.

Slavson, S.R. (1950) *Analytic Group Psychotherapy with Children, Adolescents and Adults*, Columbia University Press, New York.

Slivkin, S.E. and Bernstein, N.R. (1968) Goal directed group psychotherapy for retarded adolescents. *American Journal of Group Psychotherapy*, **22** (1), 35–45.

Smith, J. (1983) An activities approach to the treatment of mentally retarded clients in an acute psychiatric hospital. *Occupational Therapy in Mental Health*, **3** (1), 31–41.

Smith, P.S. (1979) A comparison of different methods of toilet training the mentally handicapped. *Behaviour Research and Therapy*, **17** (1), 33–43.

Smith, V.J. (1978) Psychotherapy supervision. *Conference Proceedings, Australian Association of Occupational Therapists, 1978*.

Sommer, O. and Osmond, H. (1973) Symptoms of institutional care. *Social Problems*, **8**, 254–63.

Southwark Mental Handicap Consortium (1986) *In Cambridge House and Talbot – Annual General Report, 1985–6*, Cambridge House and Talbot, London.

Sowers, J., Rusch, F.R., Connis, R.T. and Cummings, L.E. (1980) Teaching mentally retarded adults to time manage in a vocational setting. *Journal of Applied Behaviour Analysis*, **13** (1), 119–28.

Spashett, E.M. (1981) What role OT – luxury or necessity? *British Journal of Occupational Therapy* **44** (9), 288–91.

Special Interest Group – Mental Handicap (1987) *Newsletter* No.2.

Spellman, C., De Briere, T., Jarboe, D. *et al.* (1978) Pictorial instruction: training daily living skills, in *Sysematic Instruction of the Moderately and Severely Handicapped* (ed. E. Snell), Charles E. Merrill, Columbus, pp.391–411.

Spencer, D. (1987) Letter: Medical screening of people with mental handicaps. *Mental Handicap*, **15** (1), 38.

Spensley, S. (1984) Psychanalytic contributions to mental handicap. *Nursing Times*, May 9, 44–5.

Sperlinger, A. (1989) A model of staff training: the GIST process. *The British Journal of Mental Subnormality*, **35** Part 1: 68, 8–16.

Spitz, H.I., Kass, F. and Charles, E. (1980) Common mistakes made in group psychotherapy by beginning therapists. *American Journal of Psychiatry*, **137** (12), 1619–21.

Stacey, D., Doleys, D.M. Malcolm, R. (1979) Effects of social skills training in a community based programme *American Journal of Mental Deficiency* **84** (2), 152–8.

State of Victoria (1986) *Intellectually Disabled Person's Services Act*, Government Publisher, Melbourne.

Stevenson, O. (1985) The community care of frail elderly people: cooperation in health and social care *British Journal of Occupational Therapy*, **48** (10), 330–4.

Stockton, C. (1973) *Artistic Expressions in the Profoundly Retarded*, unpublished study, University of Texas at Austin.

Storm, R.H. and Willis, J.H. (1978) Small group training as an alternative to individual programmes for profoundly retarded persons. *American Journal of Mental Deficiency*, **83**, 283–8.

Sturgess, J. and Poulsen, A. (1983) The prevalence of burnout in occupational therapists. *Occupational Therapy in Mental Health*, **3** (4), 47–61.

Swain, J. and Eagle, P. (1987a) The views of parents and carers: 1. Some pleasures, stresses, and strategies. *Mental Handicap*, **15** (3), 102–4.

Swain, J. and Eagle, P. (1987b) The views of parents and carers: 2. Working with others. *Mental Handicap*, **15** (4), 152–4.

Symington, N. (1981) The psychotherapy of a subnormal patient. *British Journal of Medical Psychology*, **54** (2), 187–99.

Szymanski, L.S. (1980) Individual psychotherapy with retarded persons, in *Emotional Disorders of Mentally Retarded People* (eds L.S. Szymanski and P.E. Tanguay), University Park Press, Baltimore, pp.131–47.

Szymanski, L.S. and Rosefsky, Q.B. (1980) Group psychotherapy with retarded persons, in *Emotional Disorders of Mentally Retarded People* (eds L.S. Szymanski and P.E. Tanguay), University Park Press, Balimore pp.173–94.

Taylor, P.D. and Robinson, P. (1979) *Crossing the Road – a Guide to Teaching the Mentally Handicapped*, British Institute for Mental Handicap, Kidderminster.

Thomas, M., Felce, D., deKock, U. *et al* (1986) The activity of staff and severely and profoundly mentally handicapped adults in residential settings of different sizes. *British Journal of Mental Subnormality*, **32** (1), 82–89.

Thomas, R.L. and Howard, G.A. (1971) A treatment programme for a self destructive child. *Mental Retardation*, **9** (6), 16–21.

Thorne, F.C. (1948) cited in Clarke, D. (1984) *Help, Hospitals and the Handicapped*, Aberdeen University Press, Aberdeen, p.98.

Tiffen, J. (1968) *Purdue Pegboard*, Science Research Associates Inc., Chicago.

Timmins, N. (1986) Community care suffers waste and confusion. *The Independent*, **16** December, p.4.

Tizzard, J. (1960) Residential care of mentally handicapped children. *British Medical Journal*, **3**, 1041–46.

Tizzard, J. (1964) *Community Services for the Mentally Handicapped*, Oxford University Press, London.

Tjosvold, D. and Tjosvold, M.M. (1983) Social psychological analysis of residences for mentally retarded persons. *American Journal of Mental Deficiency*, **88** (1), 28–40.

Todman, J. (1987) Use of touch screen, concept keyboard, and adaptive software in teaching classification skills to mentally handicapped children. *International Journal of Rehabilitation Research*, **10** (1), 94–5.

Toogood, A. Emerson, E., Hughes, H. *et al.* (1988) Challenging behaviour and community services: 3. Planning individualised services. *Mental Handicap*, **16** (2), 70–74.

Towell, D. (1985) Residential needs and services, in *Mental Handicap: a Multidisciplinary Approach* (eds M. Craft, J. Bicknell and S. Hollins), Baillière Tindall, London, pp.15–23.

Trombley, C.A. and Scott, A.D. (1977) *Occupational Therapy for Physical Dysfunction*, Williams & Wilkins, Baltimore.

Tuckman, B.W. (1965) Developmental sequence in small groups. *Psychological Bulletin*, **63** (6), 384–99.

Tuckman, B.W. and Jensen, M.A. (1977) Stages of small group development revisited. *Group and Organization Studies* **2** (4), 419–27.

Turner, S.M., Hersen, M. and Bellack, A.S. (1978) Social skills training in teach pro-social behaviours in an organically impaired and retarded patient. *Journal of Behaviour Therapy and Experimental Psychiatry*, **9** (3), 253–8.

United Nations (1971) *Declaration of the Rights of Mentally Handicapped Persons*, UN, New York.

Vail, D.J. (1955) cited in Szymanski, L.S. and Rosefsky, Q.B. (1980) Group psychotherapy with retarded persons, in *Emotional Disorders of Mentally Retarded People* (eds L.S. Szymanski and P.E. Tanguay), University Park Press, Baltimore, p.174.

VALPAR Component Work Sample Services (1974) *Numbers 1–13* Valpar Corporation, Tucson, AZ.

VALPAR Component Work Sample Services (1977) *Numbers 14–16* Valpar Corporation, Tucson, AZ.

VALPAR Component Work Sample Series (1978) *Number 17 Prevocational Readiness Battery*, Valpar Corporation, Tucson, AZ.

Vaughn, M. and Shearer, A. (1986) *Mainstreaming in Massachusetts*, Centre of Studies on Integration in Education/Campaign for People with Mental Handicaps, London.

Vickerman, C. (1985) *Community Worker: the Missing Post in Community Mental Handicap Teams*, Unpublished paper, Cambridge House Mental Handicap Project, London.

Vocational information and Evaluation Work Samples (VIEWS) (1976) Jewish Employment & Vocational services, Philadelphia.

Wagner, P. and Sternheht, M. (1975) Retarded persons as 'Teachers': retarded adolescents tutoring retarded children. *American Journal of Mental Deficiency*, **79**, 674–9.

Wallender, J.L., Hubert, N.C., and Schroeder, C.S. (1983) Self care skills, in *Assessing the Mentally Retarded* (eds J.L. Matson and S.E. Breuning), Grune & Stratton, New York, pp. 209–46.

Walters, R.M. (1985) Resettlement in the community: the Priory Court development. *Mental Handicap*, **13** (1), 33–6.

Ward, L. (1984) *Planning for People: Developing a Local Service for People with a Mental Handicap*, King's Fund Centre, London.

Warren, S.A. and Burns, N.R. (1970) Crib confinement as a factor in repetitive and stereotyped behaviour in retardates. *Mental Retardation*, **8** (3), 25–8.

Watzlawick, P., Weakland, J. and Fisch, R. (1974) *Change: The Principles of Problem Formulation and Problem Resolution*, W.W. Norton, New York.

Way, M. (1985) Community care: a psychiatrist's view from Durham. *Mental Handicap*, **13** (1), 5–6.

Wehman, P. (ed.) (1981) *Competitive Employment: New Horizons for Severely Disabled Individuals*, Paul H. Brookes, Baltimore.

Wehman, P., Hill, M., Goodall, P. *et al* (1982) Job placement and follow-up of moderately and severely handicapped individuals after 3 years. *Journal of the Association for the Severely Handicapped*, **7**, 5–16.

Wehman, P. and Marchant, J.A. (1978) Improving free play skills of severely retarded children. *American Journal of Occupational Therapy*, **32** (2), 100–4.

Wehman, P., Moon, M.S. and McCarthy, P. (1986) Transition from school to adulthood for youth with severe handicaps. *Focus on Exceptional Children*, **18** (5), 1–12.

Wertheimer, A. (1985) *'Going to Work' Employment Opportunities for People with Mental Handicaps in Washington State, USA* Campaign for People with Mental Handicaps, London.

Whang, P.L., Fawcett, S.B. and Matthews, R.M. (1984) Teaching job-related social skills to learning disabled adolescents. *Analysis & Intervention in Developmental Disabilities*, **4**, 29–38.

Whelan, E. and Speake, B. (1979) *Learning to Cope*, Souvenir Press, London.

Whitman, T.L., Caponigri, V. and Mercurio, J. (1971) Reducing hyperactive behaviour in a severely retarded child. *Mental Retardation*, **9** (3), 17–19.

Wilcock, C. and Lloyd, C. (1984) *Mental Handicap Project – Grange Arts Centre Branch*, Unpublished Paper, Southwark Institute of Adult Education.

Williams, C. (1982) *Social Training Achievement Record*, British Institute of Mental Handicap, Kidderminster.

Williams, P. and Schoultz, B. (1982) *We Can Speak for Ourselves*, Souvenir Press, London.

Williams, T., Tyson, J., Keleher, R. (1989) Using mealtimes to develop interpersonal social skills in people with severe mental handicaps. *Mental Handicap*, **17** (2), 74–7.

Wilson, P.G., Cuvo, A.J. and Davis, P.K. (1986) Training a functional skill cluster: nutritious meal planning within a budget, grocery list writing and shopping. *Analysis and Intervention in Developmental Disabilities*, **6**, 179–201.

Windle, C. (1962) Progress of mental subnormals. *American Journal of Mental Deficiency*, **66** Monograph Supplement 1–180.

Wolfensberger, W. (1972) *The Principle of Normalisation in Human Services*, National Institute on Mental Retardation, Toronto.

Wolfensberger, W. (1975) *The Origin and Nature of our Institutional Models*, Human Policy Press, Syracuse, New York.

Wolfensberger, W. and Glenn, L. (1975) *Programme Analysis of Service Systems: a System for the Quantitative Evaluation of Human Services*, National Institute on Mental Retardation, Toronto.

Wright, E.C. (1982) The presentation of mental illness in mentally retarded adults. *British Journal of Psychiatry*, **141**, 496–502.

Yalom, I.D. (1975) *The Theory and Practice of Group Psychotherpy*, Basic Books, New York.

Yandot, R. and Zigler, E. (1971) Outer directedness in the problem solving of institutionalised normal and retarded children. *Developmental Psychology* **4**, 277–88.

Yeaton, W.H. and Bailey, J.S. (1979) Teaching pedestrian skills to young children: an analysis and one-year follow-up. *Journal of Applied Behaviour Analysis*, **11**, 315–20.

Zigler, E. and Williams, J. (1963) Institutionalisation and effectiveness of social reinforcement: a 3-year follow-up study. *Journal of Abnormal and Social Psychology*, **66**, 197–205.

Index

leadership style 13, *see also*
Team dynamics

Neighbours 30–1
Normalization 17, 103, 152, 179,
198
Nursing home 102

Occupational therapist
attributes in group/individual
work 147–8
general role 1
burnout 8, *see also* Burnout
community integration 179
clients with mental illness and
mental handicap 132–9
in adult education 193–4
in advocacy 194–5
in the community 1–2
in community mental handicap
team 2
in community mental health 2
in employment 186–91
influences on role in community
2–5
in local government 2
in recreation 181–2
involvement in care staff training
34–6
job description 5–7
role in housing 91–2, 93, 94
role in assessment 45–54
role in preparing clients for the
community 24–5, 44–54,
219–32
sensitivity to cultural issues
211–14
supervision and management, *see
also* Supervision
using interpreters 211, 213
work with families 207–16
with profoundly handicapped
clients 120–30
Occupational therapy
philosophy 1

Operational policy 110

Personal hygiene 76–9
bathing 77–8
personal persentation 78–9
toilet training 76–7
working in groups 78–9
Positioning, *see* Seating and
positioning
Preparation of clients, *see also*
Community integration
difficulties hindering
preparation 24–5, 39–40
active phase and O.T. tasks
24–5
community phase 25–6, *see
also* Transition shock
prior to leaving institution
23–6, 44–54, 219–32, *see
also* Case examples
profoundly handicapped clients
120
Profound mental handicap
116–29, *see also*
Assessment, Housing,
Living skills training
activities 125–9
activities and behavioural
problems 120, 122–3
activities of daily living 125,
see also Activities of daily
living
activity selection 123–5
assessment 53
admission to institution 19–20
behavioural difficulties 116–17
case examples 100, 230–2
community housing 117–18,
119–20
daytime routine in community
121–2
developing motor skills 125–8
employment 183, 190–1, *see
also* Employment
features 116